To Margie,

It was with great excitement that
I realized it was you sitting beside
me. As I wrote that I realized
that whenever I see you or
think of you I am happy
and excited. I
wish. You
love you

Joe

Many of the names and identifying details in this book have been changed.

First printing

Book design by Kathi Rota

Illustrations by Jane King herself

Galhattan Press
1337 Edgecliffe Drive, Los Angeles 90026

ISBN 0-9640300-2-0

This book is dedicated to my father: a brilliant,

witty, handsome, supremely generous man

of great integrity without whom the world would

be a far less beautiful place.

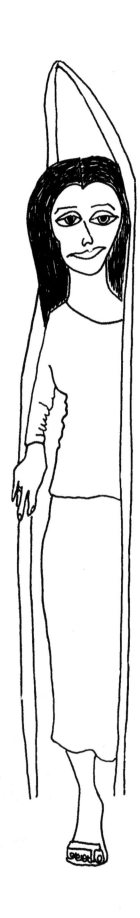

trick yourself thin.

Jane King's super
secret diet for losing
weight while still
basically eating a lot,
all the time (okay,
most the time).

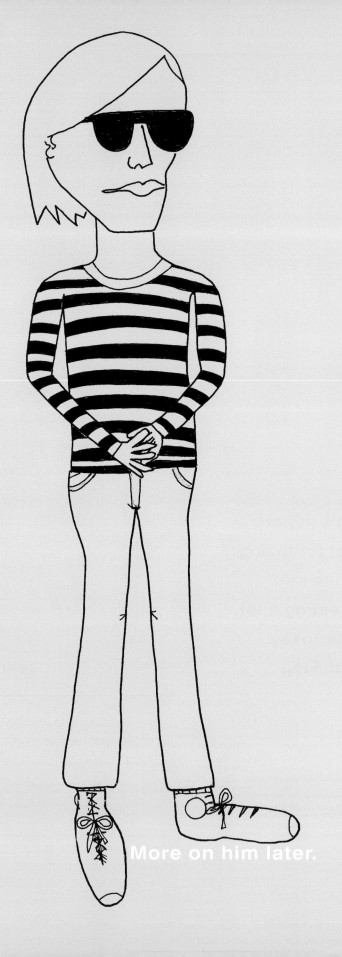

More on him later.

Thank you to Julia King, K.Rota, Greg Tebb,

Jennifer Waters, Stephen King, John King, Fred Wistow,

Sumi Sohn-Rigler, Lisa Hyman,

Julia Darst King (my inspirational mother), John Ormrod,

James and Anna Freedman, Cindi Laudati,

Paula Goodpaster, Leonie Gombrich,

Seymour Lifshlitz deYoung,

Maz and Sani, and all the other security guards at

Hartwell Cowley Ford.

WARNING

Don't start reading this book with the idea that it is going to be a normal book in any way. The author is not a nurse or a scientist, she's just an ordinary person who happened to give a lot of thought to her eating habits. She interrupts, wanders from the point, contradicts herself, doubles back and sometimes loses her train of thought completely.

She says "never weigh yourself" but every other page has a reference to an exact weight. She says don't diet, but, really, what has she done? Written a diet book.

She believes that only by embracing a meandering and sometimes confusing route can human beings reasonably cope with problems that are not necessarily capable of being solved . . . reasonably or otherwise. She believes that living in the scattered and jumbled and non-sequitor-ish world we do, the best way to BE THIN is to be happy.

Read this book like it's the story of someone's life or read it like it's fiction and maybe there will be a fact or two that will help you. But don't take it too seriously or expect it to be like other "factual" books you've read. Just read it and have a very good time.

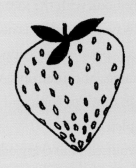

INTRODUCTION

I love food.

I think about food a lot and I am very happy when I am eating.

I love almost all food: grilled cheese sandwiches, spicy bean burritos, blue cheese, ice cream, oatmeal cookies, bacon, pancakes, granola, pastrami sandwiches, health food chocolate, broccoli sautéed with garlic, onion tarts, cream of tomato soup, tofu stir fry, hash browns, bananas, tortilla chips. All of it. Tiramisu, French fries, gazpacho, chicken vindaloo, Vietnamese spring rolls, Fettucini Alfredo, peanut butter. You name it, I love it.

But I also love being thin. I love sex and I love having men pay attention to me on the street. I love being able to move easily, and I love running my hands down my body when it's slim and I love clothes and I love the way they look on me.

These two loves are at war.

And they've always been at war. Always. But finally, after a long and arduous struggle, I think I have finally found a way for the England of my food love to peacefully co-exist with the Ireland of my slim body love.

It is a series of tactical maneuvers in which the enemy is the cleverest and most difficult to defeat person on the face of the earth – me. It wasn't easy at first. Definitely food love was winning. However, slowly, over the years, information managed to slip through enemy lines, tricks came my way, and finally a treaty was signed.

When The War Started In Earnest

One day in April of my junior year in high school, I was in the locker room taking a shower when my friend Joan came in to talk to me, took one look, gasped and literally, recoiled. And she was right. I was FAT. I had weighed myself earlier that week and the scale read 141 pounds (and let me admit, this is the first time I've told this story and included that last pound. Usually

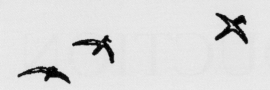

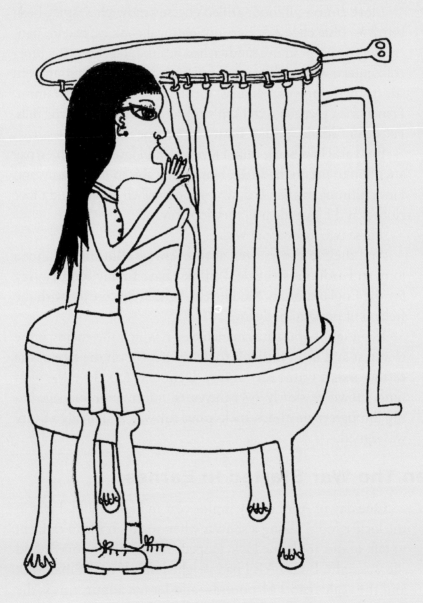

Joan takes one look and gasps in horror.

I say "140.")

Now that might not seem so bad to you, but I'm a miniscule person. I mean I have to wear giant boots to even look average size. At 110 pounds, I am *not* skinny. And my bones are *small.* An archeologist would have a tough time finding anything solid in there.

But back to the story: Joan's gasp made me realize: wow, I better do something AND FAST. So I started in on my first serious diet.

Coffee for breakfast. Vegetables for dinner, then more coffee.

My life changed. I could no longer sit through a class without having to pee a million times. I started going to the swimming pool and doing laps on Saturday mornings instead of hanging out at breakfast eating donuts. I lost weight. Then came the summer and I lost more weight. By then I was on a mission. Every day I ate about three green beans and spent the vast majority of my time at the pool. When I wasn't swimming laps, I was *running* around the water – 200, 300 times. More weight came off. First I looked less bloated, then I looked kind of good and healthy, then I looked hot. Hot. Crazy. Then I looked *really* hot and then I could wear hip-huggers. I went to a bunch of debutante parties and ay yi yi. But that's another story (which I'll write later —partially because my friend Heidi wants me to—called "Senior Year.") Suffice to say, the first time I lost a lot of weight I had a wild good time.

But when I got back to school that fall, I slowly put most of it right back on. Then lost some, then put it back on, then later when I fell in love, lost it again. Anyway, you know the story. Weight on, weight off, weight on, weight off, weight on, weight on, uh oh.

Not too far into this weight on/weight off thing, it occurred to me that often in my life I was going to have a few pounds to lose. Ugh. What a pain. And it's a pain for two reasons. First, it's a much bigger pain to lose weight than to stay the same, which means I was going to have to do some work. And second, because I knew there must be some REASON why I always put the weight back on and I was going to have to figure that out. [1]

-----

[1] If you ask yourself why you always put the weight back on and your husband comes immediately to mind: kill him. No, wait, better yet – marry him off to his secretary.

Constantly I wondered "why?" Why didn't the weight just stay off? Why did I put the weight back on? (Because really, if you think about it, staying the same weight is not that hard.) But I would try to eat reasonably and no matter how many resolutions I made, no matter how **firmly** I told myself what I was going to eat that day, I would go on a food-eating RAMPAGE. What was up with that? And sometimes it would be day after day after day. Rampage, then the next day, rampage again. I'd try to make myself eat an apple. NO, my body would eat a croissant. Heck, my body could order and eat *three* croissants before I even had a chance to notice. I would scold it. "Bad body," I would say. Then I'd calm down. "Okay, nevermind. That's all right. We'll just eat nothing but diet food for the rest of the day." But then, I'd turn my back for a moment and before I knew it, my body had eaten a Mexican meal. Imagine my surprise.

Well no. You probably don't have to imagine. The same thing might've happened to you.

I worked harder and harder at trying to figure out why my body would do this. And I knew there had to be a reason because sometimes I was effortlessly good as gold, shaking my head firmly at ice cream and reveling in a carrot stick. Sometimes weeks (well, maybe days would be more accurate, but once it was weeks) would go by in which I was no more interested in chocolate chips than I was in rappelling hand over hand across a dangerous ravine.

Then, slowly and surely, my constantly asking WHY? started to pay off. I started to figure it out.

I'm going to tell you the answers to WHY? first, and I'll tell you some stories that helped me put two and two together. I believe there are three main reasons why a person carries extra weight. After I tell you why, I'll reveal some tricks and hints that will allow you to lose weight while getting to eat *a lot* of food you like and still stay pretty thin.

How come reasons first and then technique? Because knowing *why* you eat a lot, while useful, is not something you have to do anything about.

The Answers

After many, many years, I finally figured out the three reasons why sometimes I would eat a lot and become fat. But wait. Here I must stop myself and address the question of language. "Fat." Fat is a bad word. It's condemnatory, insulting and subjective. So, let's change it to "roundish." That's what I like to think of myself as: roundish. Because that's what I am. A perfectly beautiful inflatable doll into which someone blew just a little too much air. Anyway "fat" is a depressing word and there's no sense using a word that is uncomplimentary, that would only make getting thinner more difficult.[2]

The first thing I found out was that the reasons for being roundish are quite logical and show a high level of intelligence. Just as I had suspected. I was *smart* to be fat, uh I mean roundish.

The First Reason, And This is True

The first possibility that occurred to me is that SOMETIMES I NEED PADDING BETWEEN MYSELF AND THE WORLD. And if I feel I need that padding, I go out and acquire it. When I need to keep distance between myself and the likelihood of emotional injury, I gain weight. If you've ever been treated badly, then you know that your greatest wish is to keep a barrier between you and the person who mistreated you.

If someone is harassing you at work, if your boss is nasty or you're in an uncomfortable situation, but you can't afford to get out of it, padding helps. I know some people who were treated badly as children, put on padding at that time and never took it off. They still need it. If you're super-shy, padding seems like a good idea. Think of it as **actual padding** around your body that

[2] Which reminds me. It's a good idea to say a lot of stuff to yourself like "You are really beautiful" or "You are so thin." Over and over, like when you're driving in traffic or riding the train. You know how it is. If someone says to you, "Wow, you look like you've lost some weight" you feel energized to redouble your efforts. But if someone says (the most likely candidate being your mother), "What made you think it was a good idea to leave the house in that very UNATTRACTIVE red dress?" you must immediately go directly to the grocery store and buy some comfort in the form of a bag of Doritos.

And, strangely, telling yourself you are beautiful works just as well as someone else telling you. Crazy, sure. You'd think you wouldn't believe yourself for a minute, but you do.

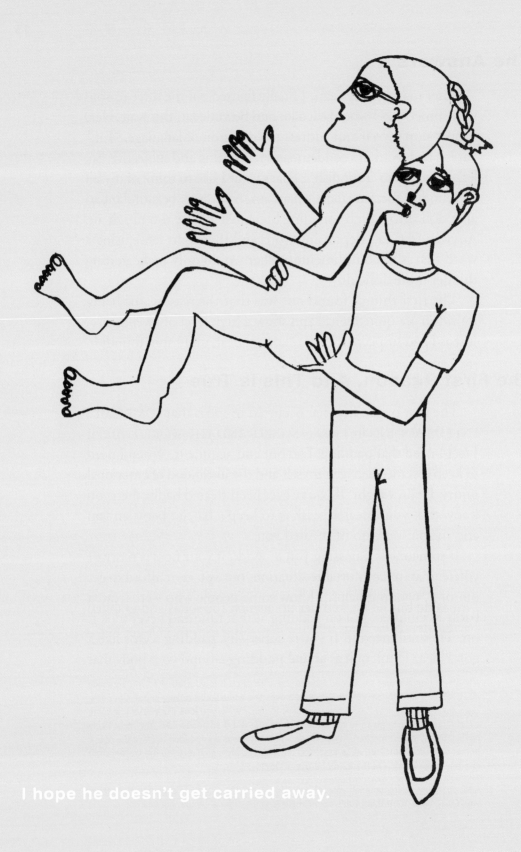

I hope he doesn't get carried away.

keeps you from harm. Roundishness makes for very good protection. Right after this first occurred to me, I ran into a perfect example.

CASE HISTORY NO.1

My friend Patty Anne is a rather roundish girl. She's very funny and she has a husband who is deeply devoted to her. So, really, what difference did it make if she carried a couple of extra pounds? But of course it mattered to her. One day she told me the story of her first job.

When she was fourteen, a just-developing teen, proud of her budding breasts and rounded hips, the father of a friend offered her a job in his neighborhood grocery. She was overjoyed because her family was hard up and her salary would make a difference. Not only could she help with the finances at home, but there would also be enough money for some clothes for herself.

As soon as she started work, however, she felt a little funny about how her employer acted. He would often put his hand on her shoulder and then leave it there a bit too long. Sometimes he looked at her funny.

Then, one day, he pushed her into the walk-in cooler and shut the door. Her memory of this event was so vivid that she recalled that she was wearing a flower print summer shirt with puffy sleeves she'd bought just the weekend before. Her boss grabbed the top and pulled it down and tore it slightly while roughly grabbing her breasts. She screamed and tried to push him aside but he backed her up against the sodas and grabbed her harder, breathing heavily. She panicked and kicked him, managing to push him aside and run out. She never told anyone what happened, but she never went back to that job again.

Later she would try to go on diets and always failed miserably because whenever she lost five or six pounds, the urge to eat would become overpowering. Being thin made her nervous. Once, after she'd lost fifteen pounds, she got up in the middle of the night. This was when she lived with her husband Frank and their two daughters, Tiffany and Rachel, in an extra-wide mobile home in a wooded trailer park outside of Flagstaff, Arizona. She had been sleeping and it was as if some inner force made her get out of bed, pull on her bathrobe and go out to the kitchen. There, she proceeded to eat an entire box of Cocoa Krispies with milk, a half a square of cheese and most of a Sara Lee Almond Streusel Coffee Cake with more milk.

By the time she finished, the sky was lightening and she went back to bed for a couple of hours before the girls woke her up to fix breakfast. The entire event was too strange for her to even feel guilty. But she'd gained back four pounds from one meal. And why?

Because she wasn't ready to lose any of her padding.

The Second Reason

Whenever I have a lot of serious work to do and **I need to be**

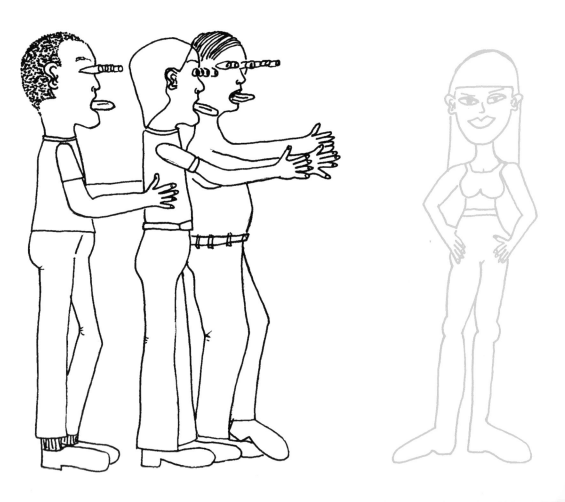

firmly grounded to the earth, I get a bit heavier. In other words, when I must be capable of handling weighty responsibilities with great reliability, it is easier if I am, literally, bigger and denser – more concrete.

I notice this in other people as well. Whenever it's important that they not be flighty or self-interested in any way, they get more SOLID. This type of roundishness often affects men who work long hours or women who have children and a demanding husband and need to be very stable in order to get everyone through complicated and difficult schedules. If you must maintain rigorous discipline, day in and day out, more weight keeps you on track.

You are the tractor, you are the bulldozer, you are the heavy earth-moving machinery.

If I lose weight and the situation I'm in remains demanding, the weight will be impossible to keep off. Without realizing why,

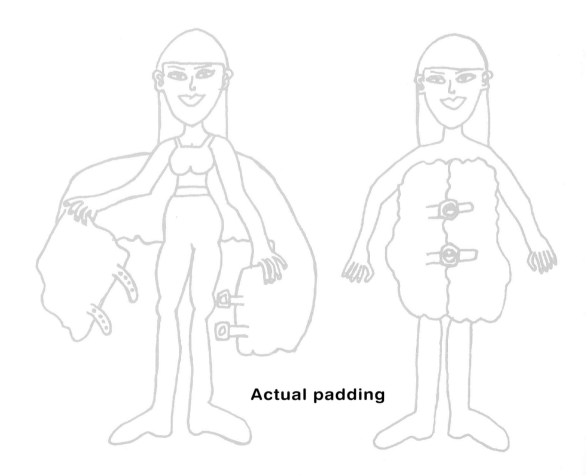

Actual padding

I always gain the ten pounds back because those ten pounds were there for a reason: they keep me safe so I can keep plodding through my activities.

Alternatively, if I become very thin, I often have a terribly anxious feeling that I might fly off the face of the earth. But then there are those times when, for whatever the reason, I am very happy and flying off the face of the earth does not worry me. Maybe I love my job and it is like going to a party and I have great friends and a lovely boyfriend. At times like these, I can be thin, because the feeling of being a balloon at the end of a string is okay. If I giddily decide to stay out all night dancing or while away an afternoon chatting with my sister on the telephone, nothing bad will happen. It's fine. [3]

The Third Reason, Which is My Favorite

This is big, very big. And it took me a long time to figure it out. But one day it came to me in a flash. The most common reason I eat too much is because I have the feeling of "not enough." And I try to fix that feeling with food. Maybe I have the feeling of "not enough" in quite a few areas—not enough affection, not enough understanding, not enough success, not enough money— and it seems like these longings will never be fulfilled. (The tragedy, of course, is that these longings *are* difficult to fulfill.)

But food is different. Here is an arena in which it is very easy to give myself enough. It's not that complicated to get enough food. Twenty dollars and a trip to the grocery store'll do it. A very easy solution, albeit temporary, to a large, and quite heart-breaking problem. As with the other two reasons for being roundish (Padding and Heavy Responsibilities), I have figured out a reasonable solution (eat a lot) to a rather complicated problem.

----

[3] You might be wondering at this point what makes me such an expert. I consider myself an expert on jobs because I've had about 250 of them (sometimes five at a time) including: waitress, writer, art director at The New York Times, landscape architect, nanny, house painter, math tutor, secretary and fork-lift operator. (Okay, I'm joking about that last one, but all the rest are true.) Also I've had quite a number of boyfriends, relationships that have lasted for varying numbers of years: 7, 5, 4.5, 3, 4, 2, 1.5 and one husband for three years. Oh right, and I've been on almost every diet: Palm Springs, Beverly Hills, Atkins, Food-Combining, The Zone, See Food. You name it, I've tried it. And I've been to a lot of universities and I've read a lot of books.

CASE HISTORY NO.2

My old boyfriend Mark is married to a woman named Wendy. Wendy was the youngest of five children by about ten years. She was clearly an accident. By the time she was born, her mother was in the throes of terminal alcoholism and by the time Wendy was five years old, she was pretty much left to fend for herself. She made her own dinners or ordered in. (She knew the number for Domino's by heart.) Early on, she learned to dress and do basic cleaning. Her mother was still able to register her for school until Wendy was eight. After that, she did even that herself. She got through high school, then, amazingly, through college and married Mark, who turned out to be a really good guy. They have one daughter, upon whom Mark dotes. He is perfectly happy to do more than half the child-rearing, has a steady job and earns enough for Wendy to stay home but she prefers to work and does. She flits from job to job, always trying to find something that will interest her. And with each new job, she's inspired for a bit, then gets frustrated or bored and is soon on to something else.

About a year ago, Wendy bought a franchise to sell bulk candy in office buildings. The idea was that she would come to an office with her little rolling cart and the receptionist would announce her arrival over the public address system and the office workers would flock to buy her candy. As with her other jobs, she was convinced this was her calling and she could make a fortune once she expanded the business and got people working for her. But then (also like her other jobs), the work turned out to be physically grueling and only slightly profitable. Her interest waned. After nine months, her interested vanished completely. By the time she began her next job—working as a manager trainee at a furniture warehouse—she had stock from the candy franchise stored all over her house. When I visited, they put me in the guest room and when I opened the closet, there were tons of huge plastic bags filled with gummi bears, kandy korn, salted cashews, gumdrops, butter balls, caramels, nougats, chocolate drops, hard candies, candy ribbon, malted milk balls. Mark took me around the entire house and showed me that every closet, every drawer, even the space below every bed was stuffed with bags and bags of candy of every imaginable variety.

About a year after that, one could not help but notice that Wendy, who had always been pretty, had lost about twenty pounds and was now movie star beautiful. "What happened?" I asked, completely impressed. "Oh, I don't know," she said vaguely. "I think I finally got tired of candy." She had satisfied her need (by getting ENOUGH for once) and it went away.

The question is: How can you reward yourself in such a way that you short-circuit the feeling of deprivation? For most of us, a house stuffed to the brim with candy is not the answer, but one of the first steps toward solving these problems is to realize they exist and think about them.

I believe that my desire for more love, more affection, more success is a sign, not of neediness, but of sensitivity. I always feel sorry for people who don't ever need to be grounded or don't ever feel like they need protection or never feel longing. To me, it's as if those people are not really alive, or maybe they are so dulled by the gigantic task of being a human being that they have simply thrown up their hands in despair.

> Oh wait, I almost forgot. A rather large subset of "not enough" is eating for comfort, eating for fun. Imagine. You have a life in which almost everything is stressful. And then you're given a break. For what? To eat. Lunch break, dinner break, snack. And the national response is: "I've got a food break. Why not make the most of it?" Pastrami sandwich or two, chocolate cake, Fritos. Or late at night, curled up watching "The Prince and the Showgirl." (And there was a girl—Marilyn Monroe—who definitely ate for some of these reasons.)

Now, even as I was figuring out WHY I eat, I also realized there was no way to make myself STOP. But simply understanding that I am eating to "have enough," gives me power.

"Is There Anything That Can Be Done?" I Asked

Many times (I mean many many many many times) I have managed to lose ten pounds. But then: lo! half a second later, I gain those ten pounds right back again. But should that be any surprise since all the reasons for being roundish are really quite sensible? I mean, is it really a good idea to lose those pounds? Without them, where would my padding be? Losing those pounds made me feel giddy and ungrounded. What if excitement about losing the weight made me feel like staying in the Rite Aid and reading *Vogue* instead of going back to my bad secretarial job? Worse, what if I felt like going dancing instead of working on my taxes for five hours?

Or what if I lost the weight and as a result became more vulnerable to the world? What would happen if someone (and this is highly likely since the world is filled with crazy angry people) takes advantage of me and I am unprotected? What if men start paying attention to me, hounding me again? What if I no longer feel safe?

CASE HISTORY NO. 3

(If that's what you can call a story about myself)

Once my friend Charlene wanted to make a small movie about me. I went on a juice fast for three days, lost weight and looked super-radiant. On the day of the shoot, I wore a black velvet dress and a lot of gold chains in a tribute to Mr. T. Quite pleased with how I looked, I arrived at Charlene's house and found her engaged in set design, so she sent me to the store for more super 8 film.

On the way back, I was out of my mind with excitement about the brilliance of what was happening to me. Standing up the road were two deeply sexy rock-star-kind-of-guys and they were smiling at me. Me! Me with the shortest legs in the world and my round alien head. Wow, I loved this! I was reveling in my moment of hot chickness when, all of a sudden, two kind of bum-ish guys lurched out of an alley, reeking of sweat and beer and lunged at me viciously, one of them grabbing my breast. The two rock stars were stricken dumb, frozen, horrified.

Were they—the skinny pretty boys—going to have to defend me against the lumpish thugs? Was it going to turn into a bloody battle in which all the joy and glamour was trampled underfoot? No. I quickly ran past the two bum-ish guys, then past the two rock stars on to safety up the street. The whole experience ended with no great tragedy. But that night, movie finished, I began the process of returning myself to dull normality – eating until I had restored enough pounds to protect me from brilliance.

So.

Keeping extra weight on is not only understandable, but totally sensible. Putting weight on does help! People do leave you alone more. You can get your work done better. You are safer.

Okay. So, Yeah, The Problem Is Still Not Fixed

So, great. I had figured out WHY I ate a lot but that did not STOP me from eating a lot. Just because I knew the reasons why I was doing what I was doing didn't mean anything changed. But here's what happened: I stopped thinking I was wrong to eat a lot. In fact, I let myself eat a lot most of the time and I discovered that the best way to eat is without punishing or disciplining myself in any way.

At the same time, slowly and surely as the years went by, fatter, thinner, fatter, thinner, I learned some tricks – techniques if you will, small ideas that worked to change me permanently. I tried them out and I was just a little bit thinner. As I perfected the techniques, a lot happened. One change was that while in my teens my weight swing was mainly between 125 and 141 (!) and, in my twenties, I swung between 120 and 135 and then, in my thirties, between 115 and 123.

When I was forty-five I contracted a strange tropical disease and suddenly lost a lot of weight without having to try at all (I went down to 95 pounds).

Yep. You heard right. A strange tropical disease. Entamoeba histolytica. You can see why I call it "the strange tropical disease" instead and in one way it was glorious: I lost about thirty pounds over a five-month period AND I ATE WHATEVER I WANTED!! Finally, I thought, finally, God has relented and

GIVEN ME THE BODY I WAS SUPPOSED TO HAVE ALL ALONG!!!!

I was very excited. People asked me my secret. They wanted to know how they too could get the strange tropical disease. But, we'll get to that story later.

In the hints to come, I will describe how, over the years, I figured out how to eat as much as I wanted of whatever I wanted, only restraining myself sometimes (when I wanted to), without gaining weight. In a sense, it's an anti-diet. It's more like a way of looking at things than a way of eating.[4]

This does not mean that the way I eat does not involve self-discipline, but everyone has self-discipline. Otherwise no one would ever have been on any diet for longer than about ten seconds. But self-discipline should be used to push you in a direction you feel like moving anyway. Imagine there's a huge, sixty-foot wave coming at you. You won't make the slightest difference to the wall of water by running down to the shore and holding out your hands and yelling, "Halt!" Instead, picture yourself riding a surfboard in the same direction as the wave. Even if you're not that good a surfer, you'll still be moving in the right direction. And if you're perfectly balanced one day and the wave is unbroken, you might ride pretty darned far. What I've done is learned to take advantage of my positive natural tendencies while tricking myself into avoiding those tendencies of mine that are harmful.

Now, Put All Thoughts Of Diet Out of Your Mind

One thing is important to understand: This is not a normal diet book. This is the story of how I figured out how NOT to go on a diet and get better results than if I did. And you will not go on a diet when you finish this book. In fact, I insist on it.

---

[4] Oh, I better warn you about something else. When I was writing this book and in fact even when I edited it, I had to eat a bit more. So please don't worry if you eat more for a while after you finish reading it. I think confronting the truth of why we eat a lot sometimes makes us sad. We do whatever we can to get through those feelings. One of the things I've learned is that it's better to just feel sad, instead of trying to cover it up with food. (But being able to just feel sad has taken me about fifteen years and a giant pile of money for therapy. And even then it only works some of the time.)

Let me repeat: it is not necessary to go on a diet. In fact, even after reading this book, I strongly suggest you continue to eat exactly as you want. You're not even allowed to go on a diet. If you try, the diet police will come to your house and arrest you for dieting because I am getting a special law passed right now that no dieting will ever be allowed again in the history of the world. People who diet will have to spend their lives in prison where they will be served the most magnificent meals seven or eight times a day. Lobster, crab, baked Alaska, watermelon, cherries jubilee, pork rolls, cheese puffs, chocolate gateau, banana smoothies, filet mignon, m&m's, strawberry shortcake, onion rings and finally, top-of-the-line-all-you-can-eat sushi. (Though considered a healthy, low-calorie alternative, sushi cannot be recommended from the food-combining standpoint).[5]

Wait. I got carried away. Forget that police and jail thing.

The Absence of Pain is Good

I do not want to be in pain. Hunger is painful. In my opinion, pain is nature's way of saying STOP. I much prefer to be relaxed and feeling pleasure. This book should give you pleasure. Keep reading it only as long as you are having a good time.

I Like to Think Of My Body As A Crazy Experiment

This point will be made over and over so prepare to hear it a lot. I am the one who lives inside my body and so only I can tell what works and what doesn't work. I think of it like this: My body is a lab and I am the scientist. I have been given a whole bunch of chemicals with which to conduct some tests and I love conducting tests.

Anyway, it's fun to think of your body as a lab. Think of yourself in one of those long white coats and a pair of Buddy Holly glasses.

What will happen to my body if I eat nothing but apples all

---

[5] You have to wait to find out about that, too.

day? What things can I do that make me feel like an Olympic athlete? Do I feel good if I eat a sprout sandwich for breakfast? Is it better for me if I have dinner at four o'clock? You'd be surprised: sometimes it's not running fifty marathons that makes me feel fantastic, it's a dinner party where the main meal is stir-fry and the other guests make me laugh my head off.

Pay attention to your experiments and tests. Observe the results.

THE HINTS

Each of the following chapters discusses one hint that helped me lose weight. When I try some new eating technique I always ask the question: Will this make me crazy? Is it easy to fit into my fabulous and sophisticated schedule of taking the bus and cleaning the house? Does my body like it? If my body doesn't like it, I discard the idea immediately. Throw it away. Simply try another.

We can never use all our knowledge every day, that's for sure, and most days begin with good intentions and are marked by a lot of eating slips.

But somehow (see the drawing of me on the book jacket) many years of applying these techniques has prevented the giantly obese girl from emerging and taking over, and allowed the slim, sophisticated, pretty girl to walk down the street. She's the one that has men rushing to fill her tires up with air, asking her to dinner at Annabel's, and, in general, trying to have sex with her (occasionally even successfully) and, okay now I'm really boasting, offering sometimes to marry her. Me. Offering sometimes to marry me.

A number of the hints are accompanied by stories about how I discovered them. And some stories that have nothing to do with eating at all. Everything is all out of order and mixed-up, but, as the preface warned you, in my opinion that's how real life works. Enjoy.

1 Start again everyday.

Every day when I get up, every single day, I determine to eat right that day. I try to keep it up for as long as I can. Okay, sometimes this means that in the middle of brushing my teeth, I remember there is a chocolate truffle in the refrigerator, but sometimes it means I eat a banana, then later some oatmeal and, for lunch, a salad. (Or I have a spinach and tomato omelette first, then the chocolate.)

Later, when I inevitably become overwhelmed with the desire to have a dinner of pizza and French fries (both deeply destructive foods from every viewpoint), that's still better than if ALL MY MEALS WERE FATTENING. For example, if I eat a muffin for breakfast, a hamburger for lunch and pizza with ice cream for dinner, that's all fattening. If I'm going to put eight pounds of food in my stomach, better if four pounds of it is non-fattening.

The other thing is that if I eat bad food on an empty stomach, it makes me feel terrible, but if I eat it after having had some good food, I don't feel so bad.

"Good food?" you ask. "Good food is *delicious*, non-fattening food," I answer. I am completely against eating food that I hate. There is always some good non-fattening food I feel like eating. Every day I ask myself, "Do you feel like cantaloupe? Raisins? What about baked potatoes?" I can have a baked potato with sunflower margarine and broccoli instead of sour cream and bacon. Or mustard and sautéed mushrooms. Or watermelon. I love watermelon. Happy are the days when I remember to eat watermelon.

Ideally, I would have a brilliant 24-hour cook who would tiptoe in each morning from his well-stocked kitchen and gently inquire, "Oh beauteous Jane, what is your pleasure, I beseech you?" And he would be smiling (because he loved me and not just because I paid him very well). If I wanted cut oats with fresh mung bean sprouts and hundred-year-old balsamic vinegar, he would go out to the kitchen and do the measuring, boiling, washing, cutting and pouring while I relaxed in bed. But such is not my life and so I have had to figure out how to get what I need to eat EASILY – and often with as little as $5 in my pocket.

Also, I never let social propriety stand in my way. If I feel like stir-fried vegetables for breakfast, I applaud myself and stir-fry them up. If I want two desserts for dinner, fine, I just speak right up and order them. I believe I should get what I want in the food department and if other people don't like it, so what? I mean, do I care if they eat only three meals a day? (An idea, by the way, that seems insane to me.) No, I do not. I let them go right ahead.

MY USE OF WORDS, LIKE "DIET"

Let me say a word or two here about my very casual use of words. For example, sometimes I talk about "being on a diet" when, in actual fact, I am never really on a diet, and, if I am, certainly never for more than about three days, and, more commonly, for about two hours.

I had a boyfriend once, a long-suffering sort, and one day while I was gabbing with my friend Marnie about my latest diet he broke into our conversation, unable to control himself, "Diet! Diet! You are always talking about being on a diet, Jane. I used to feel sorry for you but then I noticed: you eat enough to keep a SIX-FOOT FOUR, THREE HUNDRED POUND MAN alive!"

Which brings me to another point: I believe that if a particular word is a source of anxiety, my job is to overuse it unto absurdity and thereby lessen its effect. For example, in my teens, I noticed that my friends were very nervous around the word "boyfriend," so I decided to use it quite loosely. I'd call any male in whom I was even vaguely interested, "my boyfriend." Once I walked into a party and said to my friends, "Hey, see that guy leaning against the refrigerator? That's my boyfriend." They looked at the handsome dark-haired guy in a motorcycle jacket and then back at me. "Funny, Jane," they said. "He doesn't seem to know you." "Yes," I said, with the blind assurance which is my strongest, but not necessarily most attractive, trait. "That's true. He doesn't know me *yet*."

But Back to the Matter at Hand (Starting Again Every Day)

If you eat a lot one day, let it go. It is very important to understand that a person is made of what they do *most* of the time. Not every second. Don't go for every second. It's too hard. Think 51%. 51% is enough to win an election.

Here's how I eat. I eat *mainly* vegetables, and some carbs, like rice or oatmeal (or if I'm too peckish, Rye Krisps with hummus).[6] The next day I throw caution to the winds and have Thai food, cheese, almond butter on croissants, crunchy granola, and sausages. The day after that I go back to the vegetables. So you see, the 'bad foods' are not that bad and the good foods are great. So the foods that my body is using to construct itself are ALWAYS GOOD. That's a very important thing.

Because I've been applying the hints for so long, I do by now like to eat *mostly* food that is good for me. But I'm picky. The food that is good for me must also be food that *tastes* good. And everyone likes at least some foods that are healthy. Train yourself to remember. Apples. Watermelon. Chinese food. Pasta Puttanesca.

2 Food combining totally works.

Food combining is a very interesting idea which might fall out of favor in the future. Who knows? But as a way to eat a large meal and pay a tiny price, it can't be beat. Now mind you, I can only eat about six meals in a row, tops, in which I successfully use the rules of food combining (well okay, maybe four meals, or all right, even three might be it), but that's enough to make a difference.

---

[6] Lately, I've been dating someone who eats mainly protein and salads (with small amounts of potatoes) and to support him, I eat the same. I have to say it makes me feel good. Also I've tried The Perricone Prescription by Nicholas Perricone, which is a diet to make your skin look good and I have to say it has improved my skin and I've lost weight. And best of all, it's only three days long.

The girl with a curvy body
likes carbs,
the girl with a boyish body
likes protein.

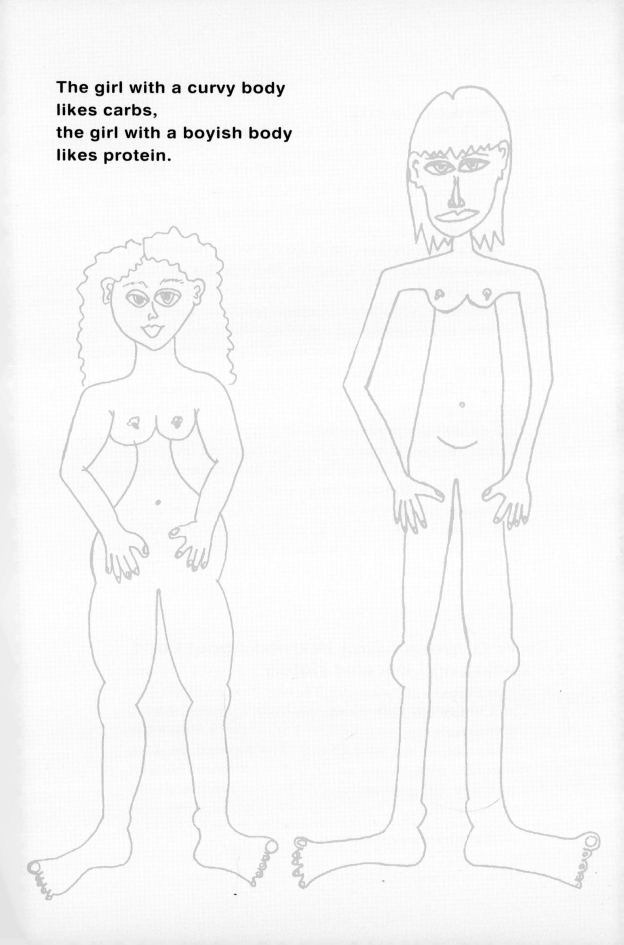

Here are the basic rules:

a. Do not eat protein and carbohydrates together.

b. Never eat fruit with any other food.

c. Vegetables can be eaten with *either* protein or carbo-hydrates.

So if you're having steak, don't have French fries with it. Have a salad, or broccoli.

If you're having pasta, don't get sauce with meat, fish or cheese – get sauce with vegetables. Don't eat fish with rice. It's really simple.

One thing I've noticed is that some people are a lot happier eating mostly protein and vegetables, while others feel better with carbohydrates and vegetables. It is possible that this is related to body type, maybe even blood type, but I don't know.[7] The best thing to do is experiment for yourself. For the most part, my tall thin friends who gain weight around the middle seem to like eating a lot of protein, whereas my friends who gain weight in their hips, thighs and breasts like carbohydrates and vegetables better. But remember, as I always say, "My friends do not a scientific sampling make."

For me, it's carbohydrates and vegetables that are essential. I need lots of carbs to keep running. A carbohydrate person doesn't need much protein. I can spend *days* without protein of any sort. But then, when I do need protein, I get a craving which tells me: Get protein *right away*. (See Hint #35, Pay Attention to Your Cravings.)[8]

A Story Of When I First Learned About Food Combining and Became Happy

I was twenty-three, living in Cleveland, reading a lot of economics books and looking for a job in the printing indus-try. In that city, the buildings were all falling down, the streets were filled with potholes most probably permanent, homeless men were selling sausages they cooked over open barrels, and

---

[7] If you want to read about eating and blood types: Eat Right For Your Type, by Peter J. D'Adamo and Catherine Whitney

[8] See footnote 5.
You can also read The Diet Cure, by Julia Ross

not so strangely, I became convinced that the country was headed for either nuclear or financial disaster. I applied for Australian citizenship. (Here you are probably wondering how I am going to bring this story back to eating, but believe you me, I can bring eating into anything, just wait.) Getting a job was proving quite difficult. The employment market was bleak: most printing company executives informed me that sales kept dwindling every quarter and there were no job openings since no one ever quit.[9]

So when I flew home to visit my family for Christmas, I was in complete despair. I draped myself lacklusterly upon the couches and slouched despondently around the house, adding immeasurably, I'm sure, to the holiday cheer. On New Year's Day, I showed my father an art project I had been working on and he piped up, "Ah yes," he said, "That's a two-color prog of a four-color print."

"How did you know that?" I asked, instantly drawn out of my Cleveland-induced torpor.

"Jane," he said reproachfully. "That's what the family business in Chicago is. Printing."

A light bulb lit up above my head.

On the plane trip to Chicago (that's right, I moved), I sat next to a guy named George.

George was an executive living in New York City who had been married for twenty years and just recently gotten divorced. He had been dating a gal (as he called her) who ran a PR firm. She was tall, naturally slender, successful and quite argumentative. George had acquired love handles in his forties and since he was quite vain, had vowed to get rid of them. (That's one thing that's amazing about men; it takes them a long time to notice that they have gotten more roundish. Unfortunately for them, fat is like cancer: it's easier to get rid of if you discover it early.) George had dieted and immediately gained another ten pounds. Then his friend Pat told him about food combining. It took about a

[9] You might be wondering about why a job in printing. I might have covered this in another book but essentially, I was worried that after the disaster and my move to Australia, I would still want to write books but all the people who knew how to run the printing presses would be out foraging for food. So I thought it best to learn how to operate the machines so I could produce a book from inception of an idea to finished product. I did it, too. I learned.

month before he got the principle down. He confessed to me that at first he'd had a difficult time eating fruit alone; he didn't understand why restaurants would put fruit garnish on your breakfast plates if it was bad for you (and here I must stop and say: ALL RESTAURANTS ARE THE ENEMIES OF FOOD COMBINING), but he worked hard, finally mastered the art of eating fruit alone, and developed a new food regime.

For breakfast he had bacon, eggs, and grapefruit juice (the one food-combining exception: grapefruit juice with eggs is some other kind of secret non-fattening miracle). For lunch he had a salad, and for dinner sometimes pasta, potato or polenta with vegetables, sometimes fish with vegetables. He found he liked eating this way better and within a couple of months he could once again fit into his high school tuxedo. (Just kidding. The tuxedo he wore to his prom was rented, of course.) By that summer, he looked good in a bathing suit and he also noticed that he had a lot more energy when playing with his kids. After six months, he had lost all the weight he needed to, but he felt so good eating this new way, it became habit.

George has kept the love handles off. And, as a side benefit, he told me, he broke up with that argumentative girlfriend and got a new happy girlfriend instead.

Naturally, George's experience meant nothing to me until I experimented on myself. Imagine my surprise when I found I could eat three helpings of pasta puttanesca without even a smidgeon of weight gain. At first I thought: heck, who needs other diets or rules? I'll just food combine for the rest of my life! But like I said, I can only food combine successfully for three or four meals in a row. I don't know why most other people are not as restless as I am, but for myself, it does seem as though the more methods I use to fight my desire to over-eat, the more likely I am to find a method that is effective AT THAT VERY MOMENT. Sure, food combining works, but it's only one of the weapons in the arsenal of my endless fight against roundishness. Other times what works might be going to the movies and having a giant box of popcorn with no butter. Or taking a bath.

Try not to eat before going to bed. 3

You will be a million times better off if you can have your main meal at least six hours before going to bed. Even five hours. (Okay, maybe if you are a man, four hours.) I think this is because if your body has time to work off most of the calories before you sleep, it cannot store them up as fat cells. Of course, it might simply be that you wake up thin because during all the hours you've been sleeping, you haven't been able to eat.

I am most successful at this when I make a really stupendous meal for my last meal of the day (which can be around four in the afternoon) and eat a lot of it. Sautéed vegetables and brown rice, for example, and sometimes with that, crackers and health food candy. I ingest quite a hefty meal, then I'm totally full and don't get that hungry again before bed. (It's possible that women are not really hungry late at night anyway.)

Every so often, I make a mistake and suddenly realize, "Oh no, I must eat again or I'll stay up tossing and turning, and there will be no way to forget that I'm hungry. Sheep will turn into lamb chops, jumping a licorice fence." When this happens, I try not to just leap out of bed for some ice cream. I have a list of non-fattening foods that will satisfy me. Soup is the best, carrots or celery are good, and so are any raw or slightly steamed vegetables. But during different points in my life, different foods have satisfied me. In North Carolina, for example, only Stouffer's Spinach Soufflé would do.

I better mention popcorn (again) here even though it takes a long time to eat. Usually when you get up from tossing and turning you want to eat something quickly and return to bed. But if you have an hour and want to engage in a lot of chewing, feed the monkey popcorn.

4 Eating vegetables is a great idea.

Vegetables.

I have always loved vegetables and now I love them even more. Vegetables are really the key to many things. Four days of nothing but vegetables (okay, and maybe a small amount of carbs, or meat if you're one of the meat people) is BRILLIANT. This food plan makes anyone's skin look fantastic. Say I'm going to meet the Queen in four days, or George Clooney has invited me to a pool party. Answer? Four days of vegetables. I swear, without the vegetables I would skulk in, hair barely brushed, scuffed up shoes, clothes wrinkled and covered in lint. Four days of vegetables and I walk tall, my outfit spectacular and my very being radiant enough to blind the sun!

C A S E   H I S T O R Y   N O . 9

(June's Skin)

I have a very good friend named June, who is a painter, travels a lot and never ever ever has more than about five dollars to her name. Like me, like many people, both men and women, she leans toward roundish and has to pay attention to what she eats. Well, one year her work was being exhibited in three art shows in one month: Santa Fe, New Mexico; Los Angeles; and New York. Because she is insane, she decided to make an impossibly difficult situation even more impossibly difficult for herself and paint different pieces for the three different shows. As you can imagine, this involved a lot *a lot* of painting. In fact, she worked between 12 and 24 hours a day and, she assures me, that is no exaggeration.

As she was getting close to the first show, she realized her eating had gone all haywire: a lot of chocolate at about midnight to keep herself going throughout the night, then granola before she went to bed in the morning to calm herself down enough to sleep. You can imagine the havoc this wreaked.

Not surprisingly, she found herself ten pounds chunkier with

A home juicer is great.

about a week left before the first show. Again, not surprisingly, she delayed doing anything about it until there were only four days left. In a total panic, she went on an all-vegetable diet for those last four days because, she figured, vegetables have so very few calories it's surprising they can be measured at all. Only a nearly calorie-free diet had any hope of saving her. Or so she thought.

On the day of the first show, she realized that not only had she lost about eight of the ten pounds but that also, wonder of wonders, her skin looked completely and totally spectacular. People were falling all over each other to tell her how great she looked. "Vegetables," she thought, applied the same four-day diet immediately before the other two shows and got the same smashing results!

Vegetables, Vegetables, Vegetables: The Food That Totally Rocks

Vegetables should be a main food all the time, not just for times of crisis. Vegetables taste good, have almost no calories (I'm sure everyone who has ever dieted for even a second is aware of the bizarre but wonderful fact that it takes more calories to eat and digest celery than it contains), and have many other health-giving properties like: cancer-prevention, efficient vitamin delivery, keeping you regular, helping you do your work well, getting small children to understand the concept of sharing, aligning your energy with the universe, preventing politicians from making laws based on greed instead of love, and, best of all, causing your mother to feel that you are a success no matter whom you marry.

But here is a big rule of mine (I'll get to how it pertains to vegetables, don't worry): don't dive headfirst into an ice-cold swimming pool.

I never ever EVER eat a food that I don't like. There are many many kinds of vegetables that I like. Artichokes. Chinese peapods. Carrots. But I don't necessarily like each and every one every day. If the only vegetable that appeals to me that day is asparagus, I will drive to the store for asparagus. Later, I might have a fondness for red peppers. There are never any days when I hate *all* vegetables, and some days I love a lot of them. Sometimes I crave broccoli. I know that I can always get great broccoli at Planet Organic off Tottenham Court Road (where really, I have to say, the cook is fantastic, producing cheap, amazing food in the heart of London and that's a feat.) If I'm in New York, I go to Angelica Kitchen, or I can always simply buy vegetables and sauté them up at home.

Start slowly. I started with broccoli in cheese sauce. Then cream of asparagus soup. Then, next thing you know, I tried vegetables sautéed with olive oil and I liked those, too.[10]

It's all about *liking* the food. Vegetable curry: delicious, good food-combining, very unfattening. Find a vegetable that you like, ween yourself off cream and butter and you will have a very useful life-long eating tool.[11]

If I don't feel like eating, I don't. 5

This is very important and extremely difficult to do. A lot of times, it seems other people are strangely desperate for me to eat. I have to say that I hate myself when I eat just because someone else wants me to. What on earth is *that* about? I mean, it's not like drinking: where the people want you to drink so when they

[10] It's not that hard. Try Vegetarian Cooking for Everyone by Deborah Madison. Or eat your veggies raw. I don't necessarily think you'll like this right away, but I eat raw green beans, peapods, asparagus, cabbage and broccoli all the time. Not only do I think the vegetables taste good, but "no cooking" means "easy to prepare." And you can't beat the way people stare at you when you're munching a stalk of broccoli on the subway.

[11] Here is a story that really has very very little to do with food but does have to do with the rhythm of stories. When I was little, I was a big fan of The Newlywed Game and watched it religiously. (Upon first discovering it on TV, I was immediately entranced and asked my mother if she and my dad had tried to get on. She was horrified. A daughter of hers suggesting a concept so low-class as exposing yourself on national TV! Although I sensed her disdain, my love for the show was undiminished.) After many viewings, I heard Bob Eubanks ask the couples a question that made me realize that what I loved more than anything else about the show was the rhythm of the sentences. He asked, "What is the smallest bird your husband has ever eaten or would hope to eat?" I was out of my mind with delight. The smallest bird your husband would ever hope to eat? What could be the possible answers? "Funny, Bob, just this morning my husband happened to mention that he would love for me to cook him a hummingbird pie."

make a total fool of themselves, you won't notice because you'll be too busy making a total fool of yourself. Are they worried that if you don't eat you might notice what a pig they are making of themselves? I don't know. [12]

It's twisted and I can't understand it because I never care whether other people eat. In fact, I can hardly think of anything that concerns me less. Perhaps I expend so much energy thinking about my own eating I haven't any energy left to care what others eat.

Also, a boyfriend or girlfriend or legal equivalent may want you to eat with them whether you're hungry or not. My new idea (untested) is either to train them to get over that or break up with them. (At first I thought "kill them" but I don't know: I've heard not all prisons have good food.) So, here's the idea: Whatever you have to do, DON'T GIVE IN TO PEER PRESSURE TO EAT. It's just *not worth it* to eat if you're not hungry.

Suppose I've had a big lunch and I don't want dinner, then **I don't have it**, even if I'm at a dinner party. One thing that works very well in this situation is to claim you have a slight stomach ache. That way it can last all night or, if you do become hungry, you can suddenly 'recover.'

The more I do this (don't eat when I don't want to even if everyone else is), the better I get at it. And, by now, my friends don't think it's weird. They've known me for a few years and have learned there is NO DANGER that I will waste away. Now if I don't want to eat, I don't have to, and I save myself from choking down a lot of meals I never wanted in the first place.

This might be the perfect place to talk about appetizers. Have you ever noticed that appetizers are often quite appealing, but main meals are the same old boring stuff? When I go to a restaurant I like to order two appetizers and no main course. Result? I don't end up stuffing myself accidentally. (Okay, stuffing myself accidentally versus stuffing myself on purpose. I know that I

---

12 Perhaps it's possible they may make a lot of mouth noises that you could notice if you weren't eating, too. I come from a long line of people on my father's side who are against mouth noises. I am against mouth noises, my father is against mouth noises, my paternal grandfather was violently against mouth noises and I can only surmise, reliably I'm sure, that my paternal great-grandfather disliked them as well.

should be put into a special camp, The Camp For People Whose Main Concerns Are Beneath Contempt, but really, I hate it when circumstances force me to eat more than I'm comfortable with almost as much as I love it when I get to eat a lot on purpose.) This two-appetizer technique has a beautiful side effect: everyone else at the table feels so sorry for you with your meager appetizers that they will generously offer you some of their food – which is ALWAYS GOOD.

Exercise is King

Exercise every day (or almost every day), even if it is a very small amount.

And Its Companion and Queen, Resting

Okay, so sometimes (like about one day a month) I decide that I actually prefer to stay in bed or perhaps I feel slightly less than par because I'm recovering from a wild party. On those days, I allow myself to do nothing. Humans do better if every now and again they spend a day lounging around, engaging in no activity more strenuous than using the remote control or turning the pages of *The Star*.

My friend Fred, who made a humongous fortune working for the largest entertainment company in the world, is a man of tremendous energy. Retired at a young age, he still gets up at six, does two hours of yoga, then starts on a round of helping people in need. He varies this

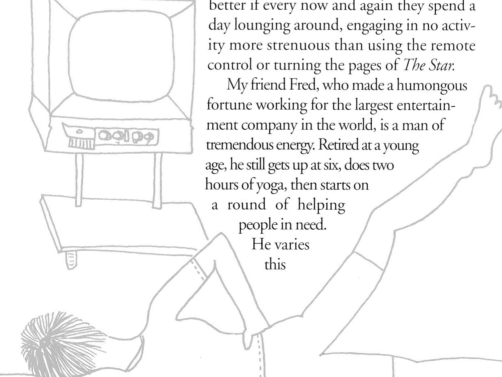

with such a plethora of social occasions that it, quite frankly, leaves me exhausted to even hear about. But even Fred, the man who works from six a.m. to twelve midnight as a retired guy, even he believes that occasionally you should spend the entire day in bed. If you can't take an entire day for this, take two half days. In the worst circumstances, pretend you are sick, even though lying is bad and to be avoided in most situations. But it's not really lying in this case because, I tell you, lack of rest *is* an emergency.

I Must Walk

Yep. Walking is a great exercise. Well, okay, walking with rocks is the best exercise because then your arms and shoulders get worked out too, but if there are no rocks handy, don't let that stop you. Walk. But never walk in an un-fun way. What kind of walking makes you forget you're walking? Shopping? Walking through a mall with a friend? Taking a hike up a hill? Walking down to the corner store for a diet soda? Walking through the streets of the city, people-watching? A holiday in Italy? Whatever kind of walking gets you up and putting one foot in front of the other without pain, that's the best kind of exercise.

There are other kinds of exercise I love. Swimming with my nephews! Since one of them prefers to run around the smaller pool as fast as he can while the other engages in a form of swimming that mimics drowning almost perfectly, I get lots of exercise when I'm at the pool with them without ever having to try.

I am completely against people forcing themselves to do things they don't want to do, unless those things might result in the accumulation of a large sum of money.[13] Nothing about exercise fits into this category.

Another good exercise is dancing. (Here I pause to wonder why most diet gurus neglect to mention dancing in their books. Perhaps it simply slips their minds.) Dancing is always good. I love to dance. I might take dance lessons soon, so I can dance

13 Just kidding. It's impossible for me to even cross the street for more money. Maybe it's because I'm too busy thinking about food to care about something unimportant like cash.

even more at weddings. For whole chunks of my life I've been thin just because it happened that I could go dancing during these times.

An Aside (Surprise, Surprise)

All right, I did think of one problem with exercise that remains unconquered. This will sound like a boast but if you knew me, you know it's actually a mental disease: I love, more than anything in the world, to be helpful. So if I am given a choice between being helpful and doing my exercises, you will find me rushing off to put my finger in a dike for sure. But I am trying to check this impulse because I know (are you listening, self?) that I cannot help others unless I am healthy myself. Is there something that would always trump exercise for you? Think it over.

LEARNING TO SAY "NO"

Which brings me to a seemingly different topic, a topic that might at first appear inappropriate in an eating book but whose rightful place here will soon become obvious. I have been trying to train myself to say "No" and even more importantly, to be able to ask for things without fearing a "No" answer. Usually I am so afraid that someone will say "NO"—so deathly, completely, tremblingly afraid—that I never ask. I've finally devised an easy and fun exercise to get over this hurdle for good. Here's what I did. I picked two people that I knew (my sister Julia and my friend Fred (yes, the very same Fred as before)) and told them both that I was going to ask them for some things and wanted them to promise that they would say "No" in advance. I explained to them that this was AN EXERCISE. Then I thought of some questions that would totally outrage them. I felt free to go wild, since I knew they would say "No". But I was sure to pick things I would actually like if they said "Yes".

Here are some examples:

FOR FRED:

1) Will you let me have your small but glamorous apartment whenever I come to New York?

2) Will you take me to all the great parties you go to even if your

girlfriend is also going?

3) Could you give me a large monetary gift every Christmas?

4) Can I call you after midnight?

5) Would it be okay if I'm fifteen or twenty minutes late whenever I see you?

FOR MY SISTER:

1) Will you give me a BMW for Christmas?

2) How about a Ferrari?

3) Can I stay at your house in LA and would it be okay if I did my
yoga late at night?

4) Maybe a Porsche?

These are just sample questions. You should make up your own and figure out which of your friends you should ask. When I did the exercise, I found that questions I knew FOR SURE were going to get a "No" answer were a better idea. Then I didn't mind it when the answer came. The more of these I asked, the less I minded a "No" response.

This exercise made me more courageous, and, quickly, too, for I only had to do the exercise once and I was no longer afraid to ask for what I wanted. Plus, it's fun. But how on God's green earth is this relevant, you may ask? Because when I learned to handle people saying "No," I was able to ask more easily and frequently for things that I needed. And when there is less of that "not enough" feeling, I crave food that much less.

The Future Beckons

Just a minute, just a minute. I must say one more thing about exercise. I *like* to exercise. Sure, it took about ten years to get there, but now my body *likes* to work, and it *likes* to be in shape. Using my body now is like having the right tool for the job. Before I embraced the exercise of day-to-day life, using my body was a bit like using a screwdriver and needle-nosed pliers to open a can of chili. Nowadays it's like having the most well-sharpened, brilliant, up-to-date electric can opener ever invented. It's pleasurable to open a can. I look forward to opening a can. I beg to open cans.

I love a crazy pattern mix.

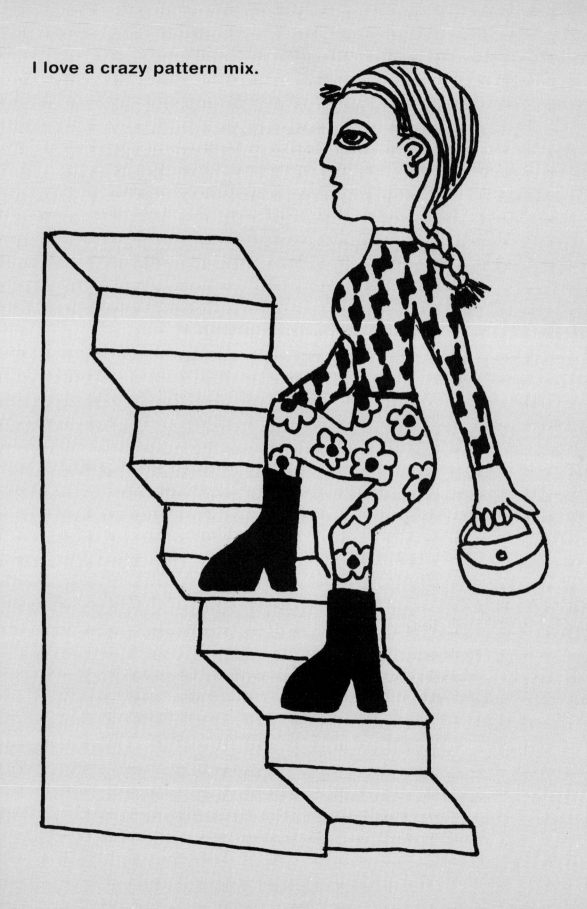

Take the exercise way instead of the resting way. Walk on the moving walkway. Walk up the escalator. Take the stairs.

And I never avoid carrying things. When there are things to be carried, I'm the first in line. One of my nicknames is "Little Janie Pack Horse." You might think the opportunity to carry things only happens every once in a while, but that's not true. And, the simple act of walking on the moving walkway or up an escalator is surprisingly frequent and that one action has changed my life.

CASE HISTORY NO.10

(Mmmm, Elliott loves ice cream)

This is the story of a guy I worked for as a temp in New York City.

Elliott was a television executive, but not in anything exciting. He reviewed contracts for U.S. shows being sold overseas to make sure the terms of the deal were favorable to his company. Elliott was married to Nancy, who worked for a non-profit organization, and they were pretty happy. They had no children and no real money problems, so there wasn't that much to fight about. Elliott loved ice cream and couldn't imagine not having a pint of it every night after dinner. He and Nancy lived in Connecticut, in an apartment on the outskirts of Greenwich and there was a really good ice cream store in a mini-mall about ten minutes drive away, so Elliott would often drive over there and get ice cream after dinner. Mocha caramel chocolate was his favorite but sometimes he had peach, sometimes chocolate chocolate chip, sometimes even Rocky Road.

Anyway, one year Elliott's firm transferred him to London and so off he and Nancy went, kind of curious about the adventure. Elliott didn't buy a car right away: it wasn't necessary to get to work and he was a little leery of the driving-on-the-wrong-side-of-the-road thing. After about six months in London, I went to visit them and Elliott was noticeably thinner. "Elliott, did you give up ice cream?" was the first question I asked. No, it turned out that Elliott had decided that when he went on the underground in London, he would always walk up or down the moving escalators. That was the only change he'd made. His eating habits were exactly the same (luckily, there was an ice cream store in his neighborhood, which, as a matter of fact, stayed open later than the one in Greenwich) and he ate exactly the same as he'd always had. Just walking up the escalator. Only difference.

The Other Side of the Coin

Just a bit of a warning about becoming obsessed with exercise, though. I have seen people who do too much weight-lifting. Too much weight-lifting will show up as strain in your face and totally ruin your looks. As you might have guessed, I myself have never really had to hold myself back from too much weight-lifting but I've seen women who really should have. Particularly when you get to be about forty, you will find that it can be ruinous. It is much better to stay a tiny bit soft.

The Other Other Side

At this point in time, my favorite exercise is yoga and it does seem to be quite amenable to girls. Even though the non-violent, non-competitive nature of yoga is not as natural for men, I would still highly recommend it (even if you are a man) because there may be no better way to engage in girl-watching. Rumor may have it that the beaches of Brazil are pretty eye-popping, but for my money a group of young fit girls in very skimpy outfits molded to their every curve, bending and twisting themselves into interesting positions, seems the dream of a lifetime for most heterosexual men.

When I first started doing yoga in New York, at Jivamukti (my only name drop in the entire book; the Courtney-Love-eating-cheese-incident in Hint #44 hardly counts since the whole point is that I *wasn't* there), it was me and a bunch of acrobats, models and gymnasts. The girls were *beyond* sexy. And later, in Santa Monica, waiting to go into a yoga class, I saw specimens of feminine flawlessness so awe-inspiring, they looked as if they were from an entirely different species. And if looks alone are not enough, these girls are very well-disposed toward men who do yoga, because men who are interested in yoga might be spiritually enlightened enough, they believe, to see them as human beings, not just the most amazingly sexy pieces of ass ever to walk the earth.

But like I said, what*ever* kind of exercise you *feel* like doing, that is the one to do. When I first moved to L.A. I got a bike and would go bike-riding at all hours of the day and night. (Bike-riding is good there because the wide, smooth sidewalks are always empty.)

Golf, scuba-diving, badminton, horse-back riding. They all work. Pick something that makes you happy. Then do it.

More Trickery, Or Perhaps It's More Like Gentle Persuasion To Go in The Right Direction

Oh, another thing about yoga (and everything else for that matter), is that I tell myself "Go ahead and go to class. You don't have to work hard today." I then envision myself doing the easy, lazy version of the stretch or lift, while everyone else will be sweating and straining. Let them kill themselves. "Just this once," I tell myself, "you can simply relax." You'd be surprised how often I can use this picture of what the exercise will be like to lure myself to class or the gym. Once there, I often change my mind and start working.

Exercise First Thing in the Morning

Every day when I get up I am convinced that today for sure I will eat perfectly. And most days I don't. Round about four I get hungry and there's nothing around, really, except, say, those croissants left over from the executive breakfast which, let's admit it, have been calling to me since ten in the morning. Then, once I've eaten a croissant (or three (I'd been thinking one but they were SO good, much better than I expected them to be)), the day is blown, so why not go on and have a hamburger with everything? At which point, well, let's not go into what happens the *rest* of that day.

But I never lose hope. The next morning when I wake up,

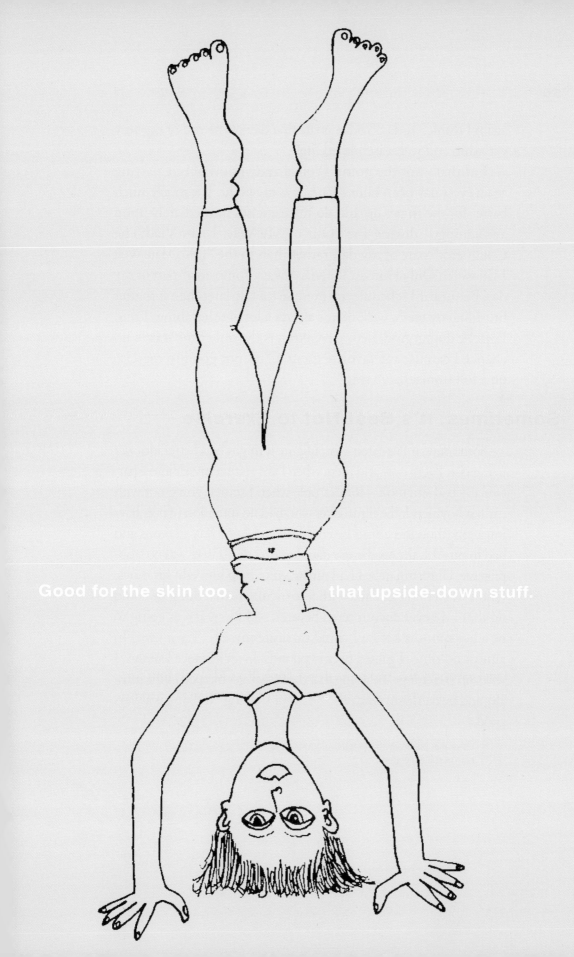

Good for the skin too,   that upside-down stuff.

again I think "Today! Today is the first day of the rest of my very very thin and well-disciplined life!"

But that's not the point. (You already know about starting again every day from Hint #1.) *Here* is my point. It is much much better for me to get up and do my exercises immediately upon awakening – during the "Out of My Way, I Am Vlad The Conqueror" part of my day, rather than in the "Oh Dear, Well I Guess I'm Only Human. There's Always Tomorrow" part of my day. Because if I schedule my exercise for any later than just after brushing my teeth, well, there's always a lot of other things I find I can be doing. And, before breakfast is the only time there's no chance I can use my favorite excuse: "It's not good to exercise on a full stomach, anyway."

Sometimes, It's Best Not to Exercise

Some days, if I've eaten a lot, I figure it might be a better idea *not* to exercise. Every now and then, when I am getting myself into a particularly bad situation – for example when I started going out with my last boyfriend, the filmmaker who had no intention of ever having a job (though I admit he could direct), I got very nervous and had to eat ALL the food every day, day after day. There was no stopping me. Unfortunately, I had promised to help him edit his movie (and I was a bit fascinated with a particular sexual thing he could do that I'd never encountered before), so I knew it was going to be a few months before I could extricate myself. (Try *a year.*) In almost no time, I gained twenty pounds. In an instance like this, I will stop exercising – believing that the fat will get trapped in the muscles and be harder to take off. [14] Except walking. Walking is always good.

[14] I hear that medically this is totally untrue, but I'm still convinced.

Anorexia is a very bad idea.

7

Let's face it, anorexia does have its appeal. And anyone who has ever succeeded in eating very little for a long period of time will tell you it is really pretty easy, because you lose your desire to eat and it's quite satisfying to see the weight fall off. But there is one GIANT problem: starving yourself will cause permanent bodily harm.

If you have ever had a friend who was seriously anorexic, particularly as a teen, you know that they are much more delicate than other people. Everyone around them thinks that they are hypochondriacs because most healthy young adults do not sprain an arm playing foosball or break a foot standing up.

Heed these following stories:

Scary Anorexia Stories

When I was in my early twenties, I had a boyfriend, who was 38, and a critically well-regarded painter who had never managed to make it commercially. (While we're on the subject of advice, let me hand some out. Don't date a painter; they're always in a bad mood.) Anyway, this painter was actually highly talented and had been very sensitive even as a child. When his parents got a divorce in his thirteenth year, he reacted by becoming anorexic, a condition which lasted for only a couple of years, but the results were catastrophic from a health standpoint.

The problem was that he had constant problems with all his major systems. He sprained his arm changing a tire. (The doctors prescribed muscle relaxants, which gave him an ulcer.) He caught colds from the least exposure. His bones, joints and muscles were all weak and easily damaged. He developed a bad back from construction work and went on disability, perhaps permanently.

A few years later, I befriended a girl who had everything going for her. Veronica was exquisitely beautiful; she could have been cast as Snow White. She had gotten a first (I'm not sure yet what this means, but I know it is the best) from Oxford in literature and had a phenomenal memory. She was also funny and quite cynical but also loving and kind. She moved gracefully, had a great love of sex and traveled often and well. But she had been a dancer in her early teens and at puberty had acquired a tendency to plump up. She was ambitious, so she'd starved herself. Now she is allergic to all kinds of things and also *breaks* quite easily. One evening we were going dancing and when she stood up, a bone in her foot broke. We spent the night in the emergency room instead. She was twenty-four at the time.

I believe that both of these people are damaged from being anorexic in their early teens.

Anorexia is not the kind of condition you want to take a chance with. Stay away from it. It's very very dangerous.[15]

8   I never try to discipline myself for more than four hours at a time.

It just leads to splurging later on. The very reason I became roundish in the first place was because I was not being treated well.

[15] It's a bit cowardly to expose myself in a footnote only, which I doubt anyone reads, but I feel compelled to mention that I was bulemic in my teens. Anyway, It's no secret. I talk about it in one of my other books, Not Quite Perfect. In my high school, everyone was bulemic. We thought it was a brilliant idea. Mind you, this was in the days before either bulemia or anorexia even had names. We thought that bulemia was miraculous, kind of like spending all your money and then, when you go to the bank, presto! It's all still there!

I don't believe that bulemia is actually about losing weight however, since it is pretty much worthless as a diet aid. Because what happens is that if you throw up all your food, you soon become hungry again. What I do think it's useful for—and if you really want to watch me climb out on a limb that some might say is already half-sawn through—here goes: it's good for keeping your diaphragm (and therefore your emotions) supple in the (Wilhelm) Reichian sense.

Meaning that I felt back then, I now sometimes feel, and, in the future will most certainly feel, deprived.

Depriving myself further won't solve the situation. This is extremely tricky and very important. When you decide to lose weight, it is much better to fix your life in such a way that you'll want to eat only when you're hungry than it is to force yourself to submit to yet another unsatisfying condition. There is only one way to win this fight permanently and it is not by forcing yourself to have only two pieces of Melba Toast when you really want four.

I can't say I have completely solved this problem, but knowing the situation exists allows me to usually avoid situations in which I *for sure* am going to feel even more deprived. I may not always be successful, but I am successful enough so that I have avoided the lurking fate of massive obesity, which believe you me, was very much waiting for me. Have you ever heard the saying "Inside every fat person, is a thin person trying to get out?" Well, inside me is a gigantically, monstrously huge person desperate to get out. Just *thinking* about it makes me want to drive quickly to the store and buy some health food chocolate.

Two Days On, One Day Off.

I have found that the best way to "diet" is to eat well for two days and then take one day off. For the first day I'm all gung ho and don't have much trouble chugging ahead. Then the second day I wake up much thinner, which makes me even more gung-ho which usually lasts until about four o'clock in the afternoon. Around that time, I talk myself out of splurging for the rest of the day by telling myself that tomorrow I can eat whatever I want. Now I've gotten through two days. The third day, of course, is easy since I eat whatever comes to mind. The hard part comes the morning of the fourth day when I have to go back to the diet, but if I succeed, I can keep this schedule up because I see that two days of eating less is not that hard.

However, sometimes it is possible to gain weight this way by eating SO MUCH on the third day that the losses of the two previous days are reversed. I try not to go hog wild (or, you know,

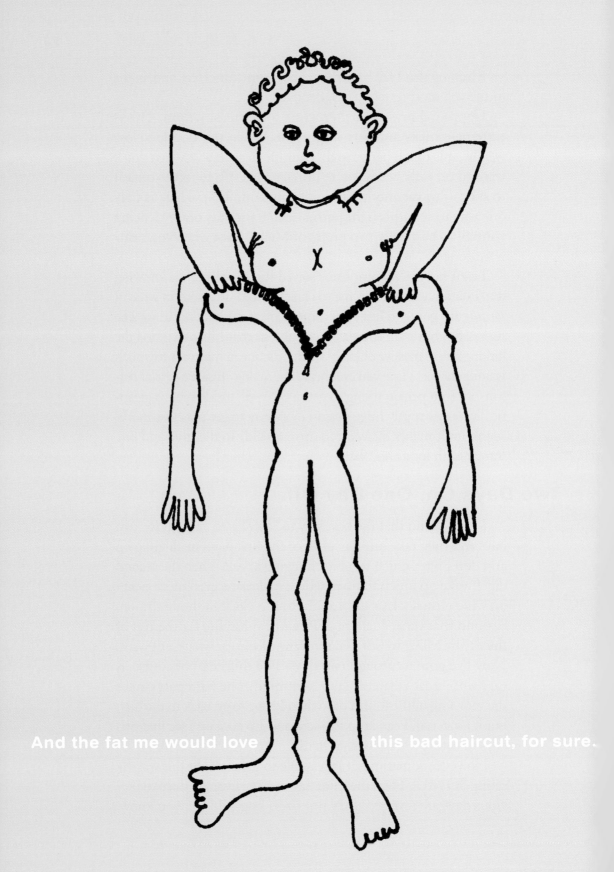

And the fat me would love   this bad haircut, for sure.

only go hog wild sometimes.)

After getting down to one of my ideal weights, it's possible to eat well for a day and a half, then 'badly' for a day and still maintain the weight I have lost.

Unless.

Unless I've allowed myself to get very BIG, like when I had the painter boyfriend, and then I stretch my two days of good eating to three or more days by using every distraction I can think of (shopping, movies, bad romance, whatever works to keep my mind off food). Hey, it took about six months and a move to another city before I got rid of that painter boyfriend weight.

Every once in a while you probably discover you are obsessed with becoming thinner and have no problem staying away from food. Well, maybe this has happened three times in my life. [16]

A Couple of Thought-Provoking Asides

Here's what I've noticed during the times when eating well was impossible. I'm sure anyone else who has ever done a lot of dieting knows that sometimes it becomes completely *easy* because you WANT to stay on your diet, you LOVE your diet. At these times, I look with disdain at those mere mortals who struggle with food. Then suddenly, unexpectedly, maple syrup-sweetened brownies walk through the door, and I once again become one of those mere mortals. While the love of the diet lasts, it's wonderful. But no matter how many times I have flown among the angels only to descend once again to the horrible abjectness of weak, undisciplined human flesh, I remain capable of being disdainful of failed dieters during those times I triumphantly abstain.

....

16 A couple of times I've had this other phenomenon occur: I've been heartbroken and haven't wanted to eat. I remember once I was completely devastated for weeks, couldn't eat, couldn't sleep and this friend of mine, Andy, came over to try to cheer me up.

"Wow, Jane, you look great."

"I'm terrible. I'm totally heartbroken."

"Oh, I'm sorry to hear that. But really. You look good. We should go out. What about tonight? Got any plans?"

Aside Number Two

It seems that my body likes things to say the same. If I have been thin for a year, my body is more likely to try to stay that way than if I have been thin for only a week. (And it will try to stay thin even if I splurge.) But if I've been fat, it will eagerly return to fatness with a handful or two of granola.

The idea that your metabolism will slow down if you starve yourself is definitely true for me. After a couple of weeks of eating well, I can eat one bean a day and not lose weight. My body thinks we are having a famine and it must save the calories like the worst crabby old miser. But when I eat sparingly for two days and then take one day off, my body will be tricked. Thinking that it's feast time and that food is plentiful, it will use up those calories willy-nilly.

9 Don't get bored.

Repeat: DO NOT get bored. Getting bored is the enemy of dieting.

The thing is: eating is always fun. It would be very difficult to think of *any* time that food is boring. (Even though I do kind of resent it when someone makes me eat when I don't want to, I am not *bored*.) So if boredom looms, your thinness is in danger.

CASE HISTORY NO.12

Maggie The Accountant Keeps Herself Amused.

Maggie got a job in the accounting division of a major hospital just north of San Francisco, in San Rafael (the town where George Lucas lives and has his studio, Skywalker Ranch). For the first couple of weeks, she was happy to have a job. Every day was exciting and filled with new information. Then, once she'd been there for a bit, she noticed a super-cute guy in charge of receivables. On Monday of her third week he stopped by her desk and asked her how long she'd been working there and jokingly proclaimed himself retarded. Frank was his name and they started

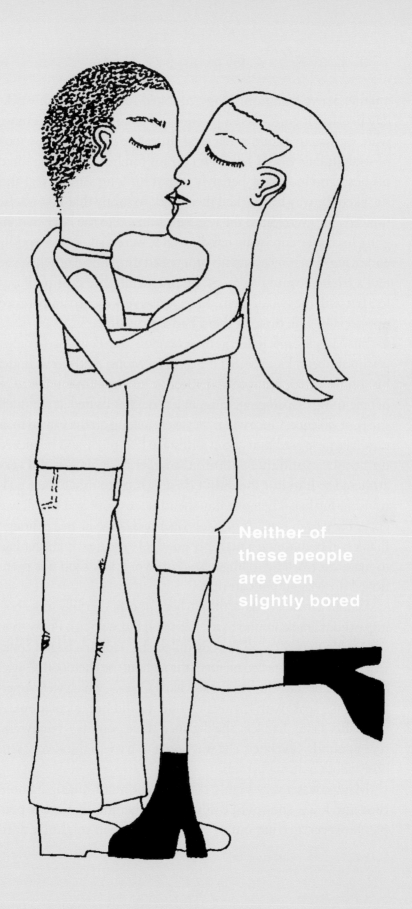

Neither of
these people
are even
slightly bored

a rather active flirtation. Maggie looked forward to each workday because it contained a plethora of encounters with Frank,
who, she had to admit, was a total cutie. She liked the way a lock
of straight hair would fall down on his forehead when he tilted
his head and looked at her slyly out of his long slanty eyes, and
she liked the way he mocked their work so subtly that no one else
noticed. She even found the way he sauntered to the kitchen dan-
gling his coffee cup by its handle as if it were a six-shooter oddly
endearing. Their relationship progressed until one day, when she
had a friend coming to town, he practically asked himself out
to a bar with the two of them. Maggie was very excited and dressed
up specially. The three of them had a great time.

But Maggie came to see, as time went on, that Frank had a rather
pessimistic bent. He expected things to go wrong. And worse, under
his sophisticated, humorous demeanor he sometimes referred to
people using disparaging slang, in a tone that hinted at a hidden
streak of violence. Once when they were talking on the way to their
cars, Maggie teased him about a mistake he'd made and he picked
up a trashcan and threw it into the street. Maggie was still very
attracted to him but she didn't do anything to move their relationship further. Then one day she came to work and Frank was
gone. He'd been fired. A new manager had come in and although
Frank had been doing a perfectly good job, the new manager had
to make his mark by rolling a head or two. Frank's job was parti-
tioned up; Maggie got part of it.

Within a matter of days, the job became exponentially more boring without Frank around to tell jokes and flirt with her. Pretty soon
she couldn't get through the day unless she bought a bag of cookies at lunch and munched on them throughout the afternoon. Ginger
Snaps were her favorite but she also liked Oreos – which were super-
fun to take apart with her teeth while she did her calculations. A
week after Frank had left, she'd gained three pounds – two weeks,
seven pounds. She knew she was going to have to think very seriously about quitting her job.

Maggie was a very highly skilled accountant during a boom
time and knew she could easily get another job. For other people, however, getting out of a boring situation might be diffi-

cult or impossible. I'm just saying "watch out." If it were me, I'd quit even if doing so might be difficult financially. (Although, I must admit, having no money *also* makes me eat a lot – my nervousness that the food will run out increases and I eat more.) But if I had children I'd probably just get fat or look for another job and if I got slightly fat in the meantime, think: that's not the end of the world. You can see this whole boredom question is quite tricky. As I said.

Sometimes when things are boring, all I can do is struggle to keep my weight gain to a minimum so that when I get into a good situation again, I don't have so much to lose. Never throw in the towel completely, that's what I always say.

Staying Amused

Another trick I use to avoid letting the boredom of life defeat me is to concentrate on some event, *an event which could definitely happen* that would be brilliant. And then I gleefully exaggerate the event's importance. That wedding on December 6th? It will be filled with witty, handsome, divorced men who have learned their lesson and already made a lot of money. Or I invent scenarios that, albeit farfetched, might might might might happen (particularly if I am thin). That charity event? If I can wear my green and purple Gaultier, I will be the belle of the ball. That job interview? The people will be spectacular and the job will be mine if I only lose three pounds. Anytime you are excited about what can happen, you won't eat.[17] Let me give you an example.

My old boyfriend Todd had been the one to decide that he didn't want to be permanently attached. (Yes, let me admit in public – I have been the dump-ee.) Anyway, after the end of our relationship, while I began wandering the world again, he started a highly successful and deeply hip advertising firm with his new very tall, very beautiful, very thin, Australian girlfriend. They were coming to London and I was going to hang out with them. Did I have any problem eating mainly vegetables in the week before they arrived? Not in the slightest.

[17] Also see Hint #21:
Set Deadlines.

More About Amusement

One thing that is killingly clear is that while losing weight is hard, maintaining weight is not nearly as hard. It may be hard to take advantage of these hints when you're 20 pounds overweight, but it's nowhere near the total torture that engulfs every waking moment if you need to take off 100 pounds.

If I needed to lose 100 pounds, here's what I would do. First of all, I'd very carefully read the introduction to this book again about why we get roundish. (And I am sorry that this will cause you pain. I'm sorry you're sad. And I know your reason for being sad is a good one.)

Secondly, ideally, if I had any extra money, I'd look around for a very entertaining young artist to hire full-time for the job of amusing me. If you could hire an artist for about ten hours a day, six days a week – and I assure you, most of them would be quite willing to work for about $300 a week, you could probably lose the weight pretty easily. Get a real artist, who's done a lot of thinking and have them tell you everything they are thinking. If they bore you, get a different artist. Because that's the point of hiring an artist, their job is to keep you amused. Being bored is a powerful enemy of slimness.

On second thought, I take back the ten hours. Best would be if they could <u>live</u> with you. Artists only need to work four hours a day so they would have plenty of time left over to be charming and dramatic. [18]

Music is another very good way of not getting bored. Dancing is not boring. I mentioned before (in Hint #6 Exercise is King) that any time I've gone out dancing a lot, I've been thin. Also, I do believe something in humans is satisfied internally by great music. When I hear great music, I don't feel like eating. You don't even have to go out. Dancing in your apartment will do the trick.

[18] Not in a position to do this? You will have to make a dramatic change in your life if you want the dramatic change of thinness. What do you dislike the most about your life as it is? Get rid of it. Whatever it is. As fast as you can.

Drink a lot of water. 10

I don't believe in drinking water when I don't want to, but I try to remember that water does exist. It is true that the more water you drink the better your skin will look. The more I got used to drinking water, the more I wanted to have. Water is very delicious. My mother thinks that sometimes when she is thirsty, her body will accidentally misinterpret the feeling as hunger so she tests things out by having water first.

Water As an Appetite Suppressant

Here's another thing: If I drink a glass of water about 15 or 20 minutes before a meal begins, I'm less likely to eat past full. Or maybe that should read: "unlikely to eat *way way way past full.*" Recently though, I read that there are certain enzymes that are never activated unless your stomach is *really* full. It makes sense. We still have our hunter/gatherer bodies and even after we invented agriculture there were still times of feast and times of famine. Our bodies are designed to work well in conditions of sometimes being very hungry and sometimes being totally stuffed.

Wait. Back to drinking water. I do tend to wander from a subject.

Definitely do not drink water when you are eating because it makes it harder for your body to digest food. And this applies to other drinks besides water, too. (Which is not about losing weight except peripherally – if you are healthy it is easier to stay on a diet. You are strong.)

Another Way Water is Useful

If I get really really hungry and there is no good-for-me[19] food around to eat, let's say I'm in the park at a concession stand and they have nothing but crisps or hot dogs (which I personally hate anyway

19 E.g., vegetables, fruits, food combined well, etc.

yep.
water.

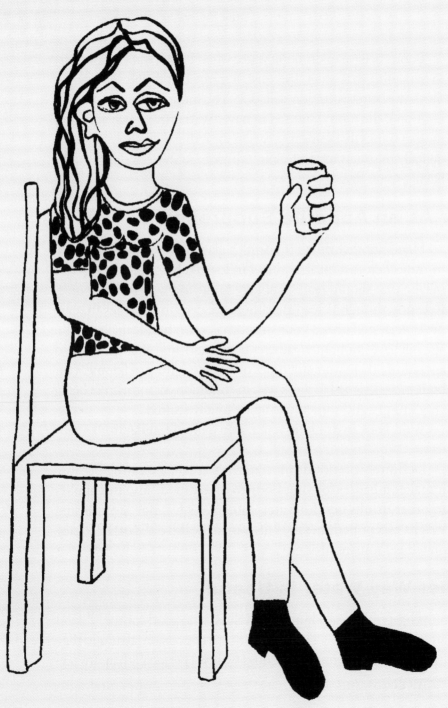

because they are associated with a traumatic teen experience) I've discovered I can have eight ounces of water which will magically postpone my hunger. Water works to keep you full for about 15 minutes. I always imagine that it's because the water pushes the sides of your stomach apart from each other, but who knows. Again, this is me. Experiment on yourself. And don't forget hot water, which in some situations is even better than cold water.

And Another Thing

Back to hot water. It's totally fun to order because everyone gets completely freaked out if you sweetly say, "I'll have a cup of hot water, please. Yes, *plain* hot water."

Once I went on a driving trip across the country with my mother, my father and my youngest sister. The reason we were taking the trip was that my mother had always harbored a dream of driving her children to college. She'd imagined herself in the passenger seat of a Ford station wagon (a car which my parents never even came close to owning), my father driving. In her mind's eye, the red-, yellow- and orange-leaved trees picturesquely lined the road as they drove their child to the small friendly campus, to be gaily greeted by an eager, fresh-faced roommate who would help make the dorm room bed and settle the child into collegiate life. In her vision, the people would be wearing argyle.

In actual fact what happened was that, amidst the melee that was the general state of our house, the first six of us simply snuck off to our first year of college without fanfare. (I might mention here that I am the oldest of seven siblings.)

When it came time for my youngest sister to go off, my mother realized: this was *her last chance.* That Julia was going to go to The Rochester Institute of Technology in upstate New York and my parents lived in California was not enough to deter my mother from fulfilling her dream. When she suggested the plan, my sister said, "I'm not going unless Jane comes with us." I can only guess that my sister's strategy was that I would provide a wild, talkative, arm-waving, smokescreen behind which any behavior of hers on the long journey would go largely unnoticed.

Inevitably, my mother and I got into a monumental fight

around Grand Junction, Colorado which involved a t-shirt with a rat on it and my mother's irreversible conviction that I wanted to use my 18-year-old sister to lure traveling salesmen into some kind of satanic trap (definitely a story for another book or if you want, you can ask me in person), but what I was getting at was that every morning for breakfast I would order "three eggs scrambled, no toast, no potatoes" accompanied by *hot water*. And every morning my father would mutter under his breath that it was like traveling with a 90-year-old lady.

But did that deter me from drinking my hot water? Not in the slightest.

11 Sleep.

It's a hundred times easier to stay on a diet if you've had enough sleep. If you sleep enough, you eat less. When you're tired, you need more fuel and guess what your body thinks of first? You guessed it: Burger King. (Diet death.)

I always try to get enough sleep.

Right. (Believe that? I've got a nice bridge in Arizona I'd like to sell you. Real cheap.)

Okay, the truth is: rarely have I been able to follow this rule, but occasionally it does happen that I have a month or two where I sleep enough. And when I do, not overeating becomes practically a breeze.

Also, one of the brilliant things about sleep is that you can't eat *while* you're sleeping. So for eight hours there is no possibility of going off your diet (the story of Patty Anne eating Sara Lee in the trailer before dawn doesn't count because she wasn't sleeping at the exact moment she was eating). So figure it out: if you sleep for eight hours instead of six, that's two extra hours a day of problem-free dieting.

> **EVEN A COMA CAN HAVE ITS BRIGHT SIDE**
> When I was in high school my friends were all reading Regency Romances. Barbara Cartland and Georgette Heyer were the two queens of this genre. I read a couple too, but soon tired of them

because basically the plots were all the same: a highborn girl, for some reason, goes to work at the home of a young dashing, but untamed Lord. In most instances he is rumored to be unprincipled. He sees her and, stricken by her great beauty (raven tresses, peaches-and-cream complexion, flaxen hair, slender limbs, that kind of thing), begins to pursue her. She is horrified, yet, much to her dismay, secretly drawn to him.

I didn't really like these books; you could pretty much predict what would happen on any given page. Say, page 217, the raven-haired heroine would be fleeing across a moor and hear the sound of thundering hoofs behind her. Glancing back in terror, she would fall and the Lord would sweep her up onto his charging steed, clutching her tightly to his manly chest.

One of these novels, though, had a stunning and clever variation: the girl, the heroine, is the daughter of a rich New York family, forced into an arranged marriage with a young Lord. The English family needs the money; the American family wants the title. The girl is enormously fat and when she walks down the aisle she is desperately shamed by what the English Lord must be thinking. At the altar, she whispers the words "I do" and instantly sinks into a coma. Six months later, she wakes up thin. "How marvelous," I thought. A coma. How effortless it would be to diet that way. And I wasn't even enormously fat. I'd probably just have to be in a coma for a couple of weeks.

The rest of the book, in case you're interested, proceeded formulaically. The girl, now thin and beautiful, decides to go to England disguised as a governess to spy on her husband and see what she thinks of him, since he no longer has any way of recognizing her. From there the formula was followed exactly. He was rumored to be unprincipled; she was fleeing across.

Staying In Bed on Purpose

Every now and then when I've eaten so much the day before that I feel like I've poisoned myself with food, I just stay in bed and pretend I'm sleeping. I eat nothing all day. Or maybe I'll get up at six p.m., have some celery and go back to bed.

And curiously (really curiously, now that I think about it), I rarely dream of overeating. You'd think something which occupies so much of my brain when I'm awake would also obsess me when I'm asleep, but no. Thank heavens for small favors.

> **USING FOOD TO REGULATE YOUR SLEEP**
> If you eat a lot you will sleep heavily; if you only eat a little you will sleep very lightly. If you need to wake up early, eat lightly.

Here's one last, sleep-related thing I like to do. If I have a very important social occasion—like, say, Dustin Hoffman's daughter's wedding—that I've gone on a strict diet for, I will get very excited and not get much sleep for days. Which causes me to look a bit haggard. In these cases, the best solution is to eat a lot of carbohydrates, particularly bread (which I think I mention someplace else is a heavy-duty soporific) on the day of the party and then take a two-hour nap. I wake up looking spectacular.

12 I always eat exactly what I want.

Okay, perhaps I don't mean this exactly. Because if I always ate exactly what I wanted, I'd be unable to fit through doors. What I mean is that over time, you can change what foods make you happy. But let me explain it the long way.

Here's How I Work It

I have a lot of conversations with myself about food. Luckily no one knows this. When I'm looking contemplative people may think I'm having thoughts about world peace or how to smooth out cultural differences between warring nations, or even creating a workable system of wealth distribution. Instead I'm thinking, "No, Jane. No, you *may not* have another cookie. One cookie is enough." Some day, I fear, my thoughts will be discovered and I'll be immediately shipped off to the camp for They Whose Minds

Are Dominated By Totally Shallow Thoughts.

But, however shallow, these internal dialogues can be turned to my advantage. I've learned to ask myself questions. Questions like: "Might I want *good* food instead of *bad* food today?" Or, "Do I *really* want chocolate for breakfast?" Often I find that the answer to that question actually is "no." Why? Because if I eat chocolate for breakfast it makes me feel badly for the whole rest of the day. "Might I prefer to have watermelon instead?" Often the answer is "yes." But sometimes the answer is that "I *really do want choco-late.*" Then I eat chocolate for breakfast and the heck with the consequences. Because I think that if what you really really want for breakfast is chocolate, don't eat celery instead.

I find it is much less fattening to eat what I want than to try substituting a giant pile of other things (which grow ever more fattening) and then in the end wind up eating the forbidden food anyway.

Oh Yes, The Phenomenon of Denial Causing Fixation on A Particular Food: A Corollary

Sometimes a particular food is offered to me and I have to say "no, thank you" because I'm on a diet that day or for some other reason and then a few hours later, I become obsessed with that food and think of little else until I can have some. Once I remember my friend Fred and I were going to a lecture and he wanted egg foo yung, but I was in a rush and said, "Let's not go hunting for it. I'm in a hurry." Naturally I was severely punished for not letting him have his egg foo yung because for three days afterwards I *longed* for egg foo yung.[20]

The beautiful thing, however, about this particularly perverse denial-leading-to-longing is that when I do get the food that I've been dreaming of, it is just as scrumptious, satisfying, and perfect as I was imagining it to be.

---

20 And, in fact, I imagine Fred will be surprised to hear, I have been punished ever since. I have become a bit obsessed with egg foo yung since that incident and, sadly, inexplicably, it is a food that is often hard to find.

13 Always eat food that tastes good.

This is connected to Hint #12: Always Eat Exactly What You Want. Food that tastes good is much better for you and less fattening than food that tastes bad. This is one of the reasons the rich are thinner than the poor. People who have no money buy bad food and then aren't satisfied, so their body, searching for something that tastes good, tells them to eat some more. A small amount of the best butter is better than a mountain of margarine.

I think food that has been altered to have less calories tastes bad and will ultimately undermine weight loss. For example, fat-free ice cream does not taste good. Simple as that. If you are going to eat something, really *eat* it, enjoy it and then the chances are you won't still want it again the next day. (Or you'll be less likely to want it again the next day. (Or at least a small, maybe miniscule, chance exists that you won't want it the next day.) But what I am doing here is making a pile of small chances that eventually might equal one large chance.)

14 It's totally worth it to go to a lot of trouble to get exactly what I want to eat.

This is related to the prior hints which are also related to each other. Combined, they tell you to: Eat Exactly What You Want, Make Sure It's Tasty and Go to a Lot of Trouble to Get It.

All right now. Cast your mind back to the story of how I was looking for a job in printing. Remember? And my Dad told me that his family owned a printing company in Chicago? And I moved there? Did I say that my uncle was the big boss? Well he was, and in an effort to avoid being accused of nepotism, he gave me the worst jobs. All of them. If someone retired who'd had a bad job, I got it. Soon I had five people's jobs and I was the second-to-worst-paid employee. (The worst-paid was the nephew of the head janitor who was a junkie. He spent most of the day in a dark corner of the warehouse floor shooting up.) Working five jobs and getting paid $11,000 a year, I was exhausted.

One day the office manager took pity on me and gave me the task of making the company's weekly bank deposits, which involved walking over to the Merchandise Mart. What I found was that if I walked very quickly, I would have an extra half hour to myself outside the office. A ritual began: on bank days I would figure out what kind of food I was desperately dying for. Cashew Chicken? There was a great Chinese place just up Dearborn. Pizza? The original Pizzeria Uno was not far away. Chocolate donuts? A shop on Erie had the most delicious chocolate donuts ever. Some of the places were a bit of a walk, but I'd speed along and get my heart's desire.

After about six months, it became apparent these excursions had two consequences. First: I **felt satisfied** because I had gotten exactly what I wanted. Second: because I had to walk fairly far, fairly quickly, I used up a lot of calories (maybe not the total amount gained, but definitely putting a dent in the number). So I was thinner and happier too. And, as you, Gentle Reader, know well, "thin" and "happy" are inextricably linked.

I find that getting exactly what I want today makes it easier for me to be on a diet tomorrow. (And it has the extra added benefit that if I go to a lot of trouble to get the right food, I've expended calories in the process.)

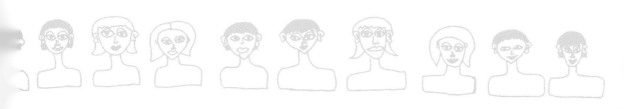

15 Try to eat in relaxing circumstances

If I sit down to eat in the most relaxing circumstances (which for me means: completely alone, book in hand), then I eat less. On the other hand, if I spend the day throwing bits of food at my yawning maw while dashing about and juggling a million glass plates on the ends of broomsticks, I can tell you not only do I eat A LOT more, but I get indigestion as well.

I discovered this concept very early on when I got a job working as a landscape architect in North Carolina. Wait. That sentence has two exaggerations. First of all, I did not really 'get' the job in the traditional sense. What happened was that one night I wanted to go out bar-hopping with my two friends, Andrew and Michael. (This story does not really reflect well on me but what can I say? It happened during my early, wild years.) They had both gotten a job working for a well-regarded landscape architect that started the next day. In a fit of pique at their refusal to join me, I declared, "Okay, I'll show you. I'll go out tonight and then tomorrow I'll work a full day with you too." So I did. And then, somehow, I ended up with that job. Which was a great job, one of my favorites. Working outside in the pine forest, digging ditches, making stone walls, carving out a more beautiful environment. Lovely, lovely job. But my point is that while I was doing so much exercise in that job, I could pretty much eat whatever I wanted every day and *still* lose weight. All was well until the time came for me to return to college. I didn't realize it at the time but I was so sad about leaving something that I loved, to return to something abhorrent, that I carried bags of candies—large bags, like you would buy for Halloween—to school with me every day and tossed Snickers and Mars bars into my mouth THE ENTIRE DAY. Suddenly I started porking back up. (And the effect on my digestion? You don't want to know.) Eventually I realized: *this was not good for me.*

Naturally I'm capable of visiting the exact same deleterious conditions upon myself when under too much pressure today, but what I try to do is not create this state of affairs accidentally. When I'm driving down the highway with a bag of scones on the seat beside me I tell myself, "No Jane, don't even open the bag until you are home in the driveway."[21]

Food made by someone who loves you is the best. 16

Once I moved with my then-husband to a loft in midtown Manhattan which had been previously occupied by a cheap costume jewelry manufacturing operation. This was a terrible horrible period of my life during which I spent weeks cleaning the floor because it was COMPLETELY COVERED WITH COSTUME JEWELRY. So much costume jewelry that it basically had to be *shoveled* out.

And that was just the first of MANY chores involved in fixing the place up: hours of sanding, knocking down walls, tearing up flooring – don't get me started or I'll have to divorce my husband again. "Nightmare" doesn't even begin to describe the endless, nearly insurmountable, obnoxious and dangerous tasks that that loft required. And it wasn't just me who worked her fingers to the bone. My sister Julia, and my friends, Charlene, Suzanne, Andrew, Adam and Steve Raymond also had to suffer. One day I came upon Andrew, Adam and Steve Raymond in the front room arguing about which one of them had done the most amount of work for me for free.

When the actual renovation was *finally* finished, I had to get three jobs to keep both the loft and my husband's business afloat.

---

[21] You might be wondering what is the second exaggeration in the first sentence of the previous paragraph. It's that the job was as a landscape architect. I actually was a grunt, who, as I said, dug ditches, carried rocks for the rock wall, planted ground cover, that sort of thing, nothing so grand as "architect."

Some people I might envy.

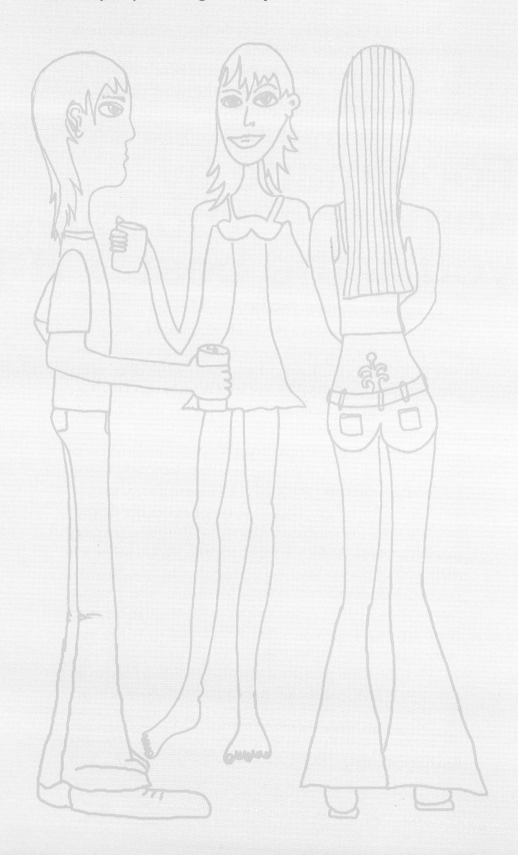

Again, nightmare. For about a year, my husband had all kinds of people working for him there, while my sister, her boyfriend and my husband's cousin all lived with us in one room (a very large room, but still).

Anyway, during this trying period, my sister Julia took it into her head that we should eat lentils every night for dinner. And it's true, we had no money and they *are* very cheap, so every night we would have a different color lentil: one night red, next night yellow, then the traditional dark green. Lentils, lentils and more lentils. It sounds bad, doesn't it? But after we'd been doing this for about three weeks, I noticed something strange: I felt *marvelous*. And it seemed everyone else felt great, too. I think it was because we were eating only food cooked by Julia who loved us. (Either that, or—and this is certainly possible—lentils are much more of a miracle food than they're cracked up to be.)

Figure out what other activities are pleasurable. 17

I made a list of these pleasures. (Making the list was pleasurable in itself, like making a list of ex-boyfriends. (And having said that, I hope I am not the only one who loves to talk and think about and revisit every triumphant episode of my entire life. Otherwise, you know, off to Camp For They Who Exhibit World Class Self-Obsession)) Sometimes all I want is **a pleasure** and eating might be the one I pick simply because it is the easiest.

Maybe I was about twenty-three when this Hint crossed my mind. I was living in Chicago; I'd just moved to Rogers Park and was walking home from a date set up by a friend of mine. The guy was a dark-haired young medical student, tall and fairly charming. That part was not bad. The bad part was that he had brought along another date. Not only was the other date prettier and taller than me, she was wearing the exact same leg warmers I was. And while, on me, the leg warmers stretched over my thighs and made them look even fatter, on her they just bunched sexily over her long shapely calves in a stylish and care-free fashion. (They didn't even reach past her knees.) After several rather dismaying hours, the two of them dropped me off at home.

It probably will come as no surprise to you to hear that as I was going in the door of my apartment, I thought, "I want something good to eat." Of course, I wasn't hungry. The three of us had just had prime rib dinner (do I need to even tell you that the thin girl, the real date, only finished half of hers?) and I was, in fact, quite stuffed. At that moment I knew that there was a big difference between actually being hungry and just *feeling like eating*.

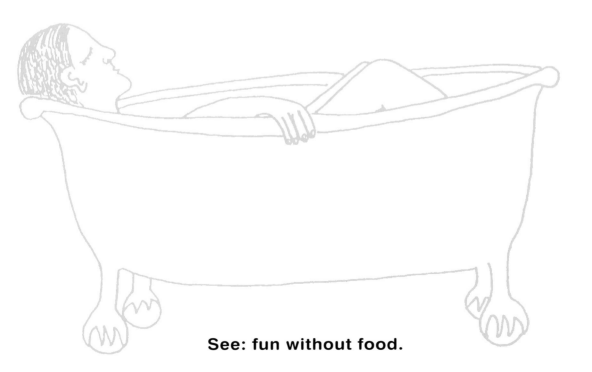

See: fun without food.

This is a hard one. This is one of my big problems, which is nowhere near being fixed. As I mentioned earlier, I often translate my body saying "I'm hungry" into "I want to overeat."

I've thought about this A LOT. How can this be fixed? I haven't solved it completely. What I try to do is *focus* on what's going on, actually consciously figure out whether it's that I *want* to eat to tranquilize myself OR whether I might *actually be* hungry. If I am hungry, can I get myself to eat a reasonable meal, like curried vegetables with brown rice? But if I feel like eating for the fun of it, not out of hunger, I ask myself, "Do I need a pleasure?" then run down the list of other pleasures to see if any of them would do the trick instead.

But before you get started, a word of warning: once or twice I have realized I just wanted comfort food, started doing something else pleasurable instead, but then caught myself eating *while* engaging in the other pleasures.

Avoid this.

SOME OF MY FAVORITE PLEASURES
Here's a list of my favorite pleasures:
a) bathing
b) e-mailing
c) reading
d) watching tv
e) driving around by myself at night listening to music
f) a beer
g) a cigarette [22]
h) coffee
i) movie

Please don't think from this list that sex does not qualify as a pleasure. It's just that sex is not easy to get simply because you're

[22] Since adding smoking to the list, I've given up cigarettes yet again. I smoked from 17 to 31. Then took them up again from 44 to 46. I met an old lady once, surviving wife of one of the Great American Painters, and she said it was okay to smoke two cigarettes a day for your entire life. She was eighty and looked great. But I don't know.

Now that it's been revealed that French fries are cancer-causing, maybe you shouldn't smoke cigarettes AND eat French Fries. Choose between them.

in the mood for a pleasure. When other people are involved, it is always complicated. And let's face it, that's not the only reason sex is complicated. However, if sex is easily available ("easily" might be the word that makes this a very very rare event), I don't hold back.

But then again, maybe it's not on the list because I hate to think I'm training myself to think of sex as a SUBSTITUTE for eating.

Cigarettes

Okay, most of the time, I think a little overeating is better than becoming addicted to cigarettes again, but about once a month, I pick cigarettes instead. And when I do, I have to admit, they are the perfect thing.

Another piece of this equation is that I have a tendency to put all these listed pleasures into the 'illicit' category. So when I am indulging in them, I am indulging myself, which is often what was needed in the first place. I guess I think of them as illicit because they involve tuning out the rest of the world.

My friend Fred has many rules and one he cites quite often (even more since he retired) is: "Pleasure is the absence of pain." And as I tell all my friends, "Have some pleasure. I can completely, totally 100% assure you, you deserve it."

18 Make a list of things that make eating a distant memory.

And they need not be pleasures. For example – driving a long distance.

Then keep the list. You don't have to jump up and start doing these things every time you feel like eating. You might be like me:

too lazy. It's just that you have the list in case some time in the future you remember you would rather do one of these things. Sometimes it happens that I don't REALLY feel like eating, it's more like there's nothing else interesting to do. (There's that boredom problem again.)

THINGS THAT MAKE ME FORGET ABOUT EATING (AND QUITE TRUTHFULLY, THIS IS THE FIRST TIME I'VE MADE SUCH A LIST)

a) lying down

b) driving in my car

c) mowing the lawn

d) talking on the telephone

e) standing around at a party with a lot of really good-looking people particularly if I look fantastic that day (okay, this is kind of rare, but still, it works)

f) walking around in a city I haven't been to before

g) fighting with my significant other (not that I'm advising starting up a fight just to prevent oneself from eating)

h) the first day of a new job

i) shopping for clothes (see Hint #25)

There are actually times when I might do one of these things and just that once, that one time, I remember not to eat an entire batch of Tollhouse Cookies.

Next, figure out which activities are most associated with eating. 19

Not that I have even the slightest intention of giving any of them up. For example, for me, eating and reading is perhaps the most pleasurable activity in which I can possibly engage, equaled only by having sex and lying around in bed with someone I deeply love. And guess which one is easier to get at a moment's notice on a Sunday afternoon?

Okay, knowing that I like to eat when I'm reading, if I want to go on a diet I go to the movies instead. I like going to the movies just as much and I don't like to eat while I'm watching. (Except sometimes popcorn, which I classify as diet food. No butter on it ever, of course, but butter on popcorn is one of the things you can easily lose your affection for. In no time at all that fake yellow squirty glob of chemicals makes you feel repulsed.)[23]

Reading and Eating Will Always Make Me Happy. Always

When I was young, reading and eating at the same time was my top favorite thing. (And may still be.) One of the worst parts of growing up was that I was not allowed to read while eating lunch at school or during dinner at home. So I would have to sit during these meals, the cacophony of six brothers and sisters swirling around the table, with my current favorite book, secretly open, on my lap.

I do find that it is possible for me to read without eating if I lie down. Even on a couch.

Or sometimes I give up reading for a week.

20 Postpone eating.

This is a technique that all the really skinny girls in New York use, especially the ones that work for the magazines.

....

23 Now I've given up popcorn, too. The strange tropical disease I had (see Hint #32) made eating it hurt my insides. Just in the nick of time, too, since I am in love with a guy who hates people who eat popcorn. STOP READING HERE IF YOU HATE OBSESSION OR CRAZY TANGENTS (even though I warned you about this very thing in the preface). Okay, maybe it's not such a good thing I stopped eating popcorn from that standpoint because it's a bad romance and I'm pretty sure the guy doesn't love me because he hates blondes (or maybe I'm not pretty enough). But on the other hand (I mean very much the other hand, so much so that maybe it's the other hand on a whole other person) it's still good I gave up popcorn and quite surprisingly I didn't become fat when I did.

Which reminds me of something else: how the deeply rich stay thin. My friend Hunter took me to "21" and asked if he could do all the ordering. "Sure," I said. Hunter is tall, blonde and quite thin himself, partial to Armani suits. Very English-looking. (To tell you the truth, I'm not enamored of those super-tall guys. I mean, I can wear the highest shoes in the world and stand up straight but then, after I go to all that effort, I like to be close in height to them. To me it's just not sexy when someone has to lean WAY over to hug you. I know it's not their fault, but still.)

Anyway there we were at "21" and Hunter ordered a meal with appetizer, soup, salad and entrée. When my Portobello mushroom tart drizzled with truffle compote arrived, I was delighted and totally scarfed it. (Except for the bite I politely offered to Hunter, of course.) It was delicious. As was my Lobster Bisque. And the pear, candied pecans and Gorgonzola salad. But by then I was feeling a little full and really could have skipped the peppered filet with garlic and leek mashed potatoes.

"How can the rich women eat so much and still stay thin?" I asked Hunter.

He leaned across the table in his elegant way, smiling ever so slightly. "They only eat a small amount of each course."

Ah ha! I thought. *That's* how they do it. Not that that would be possible for me, because I know that not eating all your food is a mortal sin. In fact, I'm pretty sure I learned that leaving food on your plate was a sin long before I learned of the existence of God. But the concept is good. Just don't prepare (or order) too much food to start with.

But curiously enough, I have once again strayed from the subject matter.

And That Subject Was, I Believe, Postponement

Try to be careful not to postpone eating only to have a big pigout at midnight, seconds before you go to bed.

Try to postpone a meal by 15 minutes.

Try to embrace the idea of being slightly hungry.

Frank, If You're Out There, I Still Think Of You

There was a guy I met in Chicago named Frank Rothschild who was quite thin. He once told me he always ate less than he wanted because he so much loved the feeling of being hungry.[24]

To my mind, this is going too far and it would be impossible to seriously date someone who felt this way, but the idea should be considered. I've been trying not to hate the feeling of being hungry quite so much. To hate it slightly less. To tease myself by allowing it to stay for a couple of minutes. Look at it. What's it like? It *is* hateful, but still this exercise is worth doing.

This is a lot like when naturally thin people say, "Wow, I forgot to eat."

This is completely astounding to me. Forgot to *eat*? Please. Forgot to call the dentist, sure. Forgot to do the dishes? Yes. Forgot to brush my hair? Forgot to go to work? Maybe. Forgot my boyfriend's name? Possible. But forgot to eat? No. Maybe once, a long time ago and I'm sure even that was only for about three hours. But not a *whole* day. Forgot to <u>eat</u>? What could they be they thinking? That is a person from another planet.

How I Talk To Myself

So postponing is good, but not always possible. Here is an example: this morning, I had a banana for breakfast and then I was going to have a brioche after the banana had been digested. But since I had already bought the brioche and it was sitting there waiting for me, it was nearly impossible to postpone. "Okay," I said to myself. "You only have to postpone eating the brioche for one hour."

So how do I occupy myself while I am postponing? Well, I can exercise, watch tv, type a letter, clean the bathroom, all mentioned because, in actual fact, I did these things just this morning. So then an hour does go by and I pull out the brioche. And . . . just before I remove it from its white paper bag (it is *so* beautiful, that bulbous shape and those sections, that melt-in-your

24 And by the way, Frank lived in an all-black apartment of such stunning spotlessness that my first question upon entering was "Do you have a cleaning lady?" because if he said "no," I was so totally out of there. (He said "yes." But I still don't know if he was telling the truth.)

mouth-ness. Oh lovely. Lovely. I want another right now, just thinking about it.) I try to talk myself into waiting fifteen minutes more. No way. I can't. I rip open the bag and take the first big, buttery, satisfying bite.

So what I've learned is that I can postpone eating, but not for one minute longer than I told myself in my initial bargain.

This is true in other areas, too. I can do a certain amount of work I find particularly obnoxious by telling myself that I only have to do it for an hour. But then at the end of that hour, I cannot trick myself into postponing yet again. (This is a perfect example of *tricking*, not *lying*.) But when I stop, I want to have a pleasure. Which brings us to the point of using food for other gains:

I use food constantly as a carrot; I promise myself some food item if I finish a chore. But I try to save this for only the worst chores and, if I'm getting too fat doing this, then I know that my life has gotten too tedious and needs to be adjusted.

Some Other Thoughts, Not Really About Postponing

Roundishness is also an early warning signal, like a canary in a mine. If I start getting too roundish, that's a sure sign I'm not happy in my life. Something must change. Do I hate where I live? Am I driving in traffic too much? Do I have a bad boyfriend? Am I fooling myself that he treats me well? As you might have noticed, I've had plenty of boyfriends in my life and I know that when one treats me well, I lose weight.[25] What about my job? Am I being abused? Because jobs work exactly the same as boyfriends: when I'm being treated well, the weight falls off.

My feeling is that whether or not we have other lives, this one MUST be filled with joy. If you are the sort who doesn't believe it's imperative to have a good time, remember, it is hard for the people around you to have a good time if you're having a bad time. Have you no obligation to them?

....

[25] And okay, I'm sure I sound like a maniac, but I cannot emphasize enough that a bad boyfriend is a primary reason for getting too roundish, so WATCH OUT for bad boyfriends and bad husbands!

Oh, another good thing about postponing is that every once in a great while, when I get to the appointed hour, I lose my desire to overeat. Granted this happens only rarely, but remember, we're building a wall here and every brick counts.

21 Set deadlines.

This is another way I talk myself into temporarily eating less.

I invent the idea that some event in the immediate future necessitates that I be thinner than I currently am. My thinness is of desperate—nay, critical—importance. For example, if I am going to a party on Saturday, I convince myself that my future true love will be there for sure but his only flaw is an inability to be attracted to women unless they are four pounds thinner than I am right this minute. (Later, I will break him of this ill-conceived notion, but first I must get my foot in the door.) This ploy gives me the energy and motivation to diet rigorously for a couple of days. And it does not involve lying. (As you know by now, I am very much opposed to lying.) Although it is far-fetched that my future true love will be there, hey, anything is possible. The more I expect extraordinary things, the more they actually happen.

But, I must also be careful not to go too far. As my friend Lisa says, "Oh yeah, at any wedding you can look around and spot the girls who no longer fill out their bustline and you think, 'Someone get that girl a dessert quick!'"

When the nuptials for which I have struggled so mightily to lose weight have come and gone, I set my sights on some other event in the very near future. After setting a few deadlines like this, I saw that most of the "events" turn out to be tragically uneventful, so I only diet for a couple of days, thus avoiding needless torture for too many days. Job interview this week? I eat lightly for two days. Party on Friday? Two days. First day of work Monday? That's an easy one. Never eat the first day on a new job, it gives you indigestion. See? If you do this on a day-by-day basis, you never give up, you never work too hard and you never make yourself feel bad for failing. You just pick yourself up and get back on the horse. This is a life long process, not just for a week or a day.

Plus, It's Fun to Exaggerate

One of the more amusing side benefits of this technique is that if I go to a dinner before a big event and I only nibble on cauliflower and broccoli while everyone else gobbles down incredibly delicious chicken casserole (and, geez, just typing those words makes my mouth water), then, if, say, I'm sitting next to some guy who asks, "Aren't you hungry?" I can respond by saying, "I can't eat a thing. I have to lose a lot of weight because I am going to meet my next boyfriend at this party I'm attending tomorrow night." The guy will think it's a laugh riot that I expect to lose a lot of weight overnight. If I add that I am hoping to lose at least fifteen pounds in the next 24 hours, he will really laugh, if for no other reason than that it is such a stunning example of how much different girls are from boys.

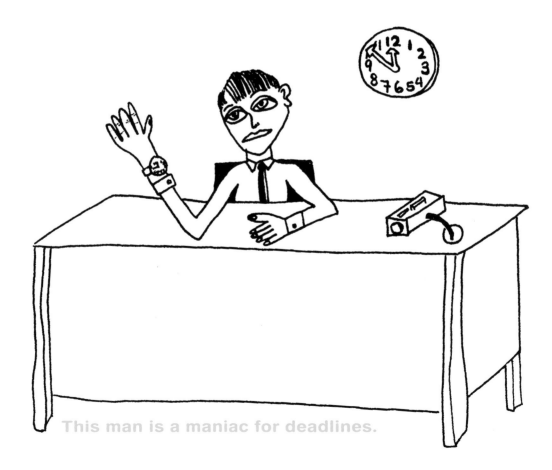

This man is a maniac for deadlines.

And My Experience?

Sometimes setting a deadline works. Sometimes you ARE really happy you are three pounds thinner. Sometimes the event *is* every bit as exciting and glamorous as you thought it would be and the loss of those few extra pounds allows you to blindingly shine.

The Most Amazing Wedding

On the other hand, here's a perfect story about losing too much weight for an event that ends up having a happy ending anyway. Well, of course, in one sense, is there really any such thing as losing *too much* weight, short of being anorexic? The two times I was ever really thin in my life all my friends wanted to take me out to eat, which I totally loved for many reasons. Unfortunately, I said yes to all the invitations and so the weight reattached itself in no time, but, oh, how glorious were those times of total thinness. (Oh hmm, yes. And the time of the strange tropical disease when it was a bit scary how thin I was. That was definitely too much weight lost.)

Anyway. Many many years ago, I was asked to be a bridesmaid in the wedding of a girl who worked with me in Chicago. I was very excited because this wedding promised to be interesting: he was a big drug dealer and she was a cocaine addict. When they hooked up, she had access to so much of her drug of choice she started having cocaine-induced epileptic seizures at the grocery store. A few minutes after she'd go out to buy milk, he would hear ambulance sirens and know they were for her.

Well, the dealer was not a calloused sort. He actually loved her and paid for her to go to rehab in a small town nestled beside the train tracks somewhere in the flat, dusty Midwest.

Months went by. She did well in rehab and near the end of her stay, there was a Saturday night dance at the clinic. He came, they stayed in a motel and her body—probably deeply relieved at being clean, immediately became pregnant. They decided to marry.

I was living in another state and it was not possible for me to be measured for my bridesmaid dress in advance so I lied (Oh. Ummm. I mean, "projected into the future") and phoned in smaller measurements thinking that that would force me to trick myself thin by the time of the event. Immediately I panicked, thinking of how embarrassing it would be for me to have to have my dress ENLARGED at the last minute, so I ate very little.

Meanwhile, back in her hometown of Grosse Pointe, the bride was a bit at a loss as to whom to invite to her wedding and further, who else could she ask to be bridesmaids. All her old friends were still drug addicts, so she decided to ask the girls with whom she'd been in rehab. Well, the week of the very large, very social event arrived. (Did I say that both came from socially prominent families and the drug dealer was quite quite wealthy from his profession?) I traveled to their town, tried on the dress and found I had been more than successful. My dress was now enormous; I could barely keep it on. I kind of liked the feeling, so I prevented the seamstress from taking it in.

As soon as I got there, I could tell that the festivities were going to turn out to be every bit as extraordinary as I had expected. The rehabbed bridesmaids were beautiful, quite savage, and, it seemed, wanton beyond belief. Many of them were staying in the country mansion of the groom's family and were sleeping with the groom's handsome younger brothers and generally running wild through the many oriental rug-covered halls.

On the day of the wedding, I slipped into my gown (and almost back out the other side) and proceeded to swim around inside the peach silk material in a way that might not have looked so fetching, but felt tremendously satisfying. And most amusingly, the slatternly complement of bridesmaids, deeply jealous that the sleeves fell so enticingly off my shoulders, all pulled their sleeves off their shoulders as well.

The bride wore a jewel-encrusted gown. It was a beautiful sunny day. Everyone wore sunglasses and it was a fantastic, amazing, surreal experience, like being in a Lina Wertmuller film.

22 Take some foods that are normally thought of as diet foods and imagine that they are forbidden.

Bananas, watermelon, plain bread with margarine, wheat thins. Don't *ever* allow yourself to eat these things when you're on a diet. Then, when you really want to binge, eat a banana or a giant slice of watermelon, feel totally guilty, bemoan the fact that you have failed to stay on your diet, only to find the next day: SURPRISE, SURPRISE! You are not rounder, you are just about the same size!!

23 Sometimes eating is just about the fun of chewing and swallowing.

Years ago, I realized that what I really really liked about eating (oh, I do hope no normal people are reading this book, because this is going to sound severely weird) was chewing and swallowing. I mean, I like food in my mouth and I definitely like the taste of food and I also love the feeling of a full stomach. (At least at first. Later I'm forced to recognize yet again that "full stomach" today = "roundish" tomorrow, and that part I *don't* like.)

But the thing I like the <u>most</u> is chewing and swallowing. Which I guess is partly about the taste of food. It took me a long time to figure this out.

CASE HISTORY NO.13

Peg is an avid reader of romance novels. Nothing makes her happier than to curl up on a soft couch with a blanket, read a novel and eat (like me). When she was younger, she ate mainly chocolate and chips (Snickers bars and BBQ potato chips were her favorites), but then she slowly developed a fondness for popcorn, which—as was pointed out earlier—is a non-fattening food that one can eat for hours, and now she usually settles in with popcorn and a bag of pre-washed organic spinach.

Sounds impossible, right? Also insane? But no, it's true. Now she actually *prefers* the fresh green taste of spinach to greasy potato chips and overly-sweet candy bars. And the point for her really is to eat a food you can slowly reach for, doesn't muck up the blanket or couch if you drop it, and that you can eat for a long, long time. Sometimes she has spinach first, sometimes popcorn first. When she is totally full, she snuggles down further into the soft couch and by the time she's gotten to the juicy bits of the book, she's happy. If she happens to drift off, when she wakes up in the morning she still loves herself, because the food she's eaten has used up (almost) more calories getting digested than it contained in the first place. Brilliant, Peg. Utterly brilliant.

Sometimes she does still have chocolate and chips, but if she has five reading-and-eating evenings in a month (which is more likely now that her youngest has gone off to college and her husband plays poker with some other self-designated bigwigs), the snacks on three of these nights are spinach and popcorn and only on two does she devour chocolate and chips.

24. Don't drink any-thing with calories.

Let's face it, my life has been a bit of a madhouse. I've wanted to have a lot of experiences and I certainly got them. Partially because, if I am given a choice between two alternatives, I like to choose the odder one, the one where I don't know the outcome. But because of this, I often find myself in situations which, quite frankly, are beyond me. Often it takes years for me to figure out what's going on. Many many many years.

So it certainly wasn't in one blinding aha! moment that I realized that it was the act of chewing that I liked so much or that calories in drink were no longer worth it. No. These, like most insights and understandings, were the product of a very slow awakening. It wasn't that I didn't *like* the taste of hot chocolate or Coke. No, it was that I liked the taste (and chewing and swallowing) of chocolate and candy bars *so much* that *drinking* my calories seemed a senseless waste. Now I basically drink only water and take all my calories in solid form.

I used to drink Diet Coke, which had a pretty good taste. I really liked how, after I would eat a lot, a Diet Coke acted kind of magically: the bubbles would push my stomach out just a little bit more, then they'd be gone, and that process would somehow make me more comfortable after a meal that had verged on the excessive. I loved that. (I used to buy cases of Diet Coke and store them vertically in my locker at school.)

But when they published the findings that saccharine causes irreparable damage to the brains of unborn fetuses,[26] I had no trouble giving up Diet Coke. First of all, it's not *that* good, and second of all, I didn't see that my brain was so very much different than the brain of an unborn fetus. We are talking the same species. Scary.

....

26 You know, I THINK I read this. But is was SO long ago. But why take a chance?

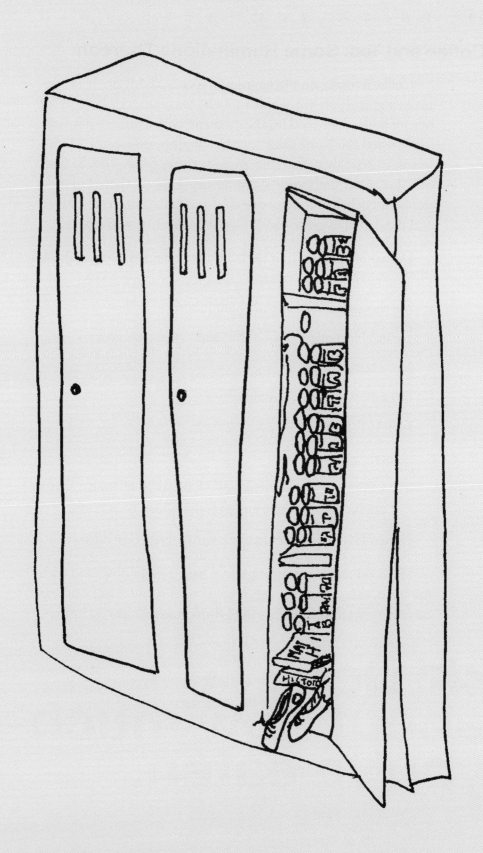

Coffee and Tea: Some Ruminations Thereon

Coffee is totally non-fattening and speeds a body up. It's sometimes a great high but seems to make you hungrier later. A lot of stuff is like that: good for the moment, with a price to pay later. Caffeinated tea? Same thing, maybe a slightly lesser price. Herbal teas don't have this effect and are sometimes good. They're basically hot water with some slight flavoring, aren't they? I used to drink a lot of herbal teas but one day I was having my teeth cleaned and the dental hygienist and I had the following conversation:

Dental Hygienist: Your teeth are a little stained. Do you drink coffee?

Me (horrified)(and slightly lying): No!

Dental Hygienist: What about tea?

Me: Herbal Tea.

Dental Hygienist: Tea stains your teeth.

Me: ALL TEA?!??!!

Dental Hygienist: Yes.

Me: Oh my God. I didn't know. (Extremely agitated.) What about food? Is there any *food* that stains your teeth?

Dental Hygienist (very firmly): Curry. Never eat curry.

Since, on top of everything else, I have a slight obsession with my teeth, this conversation produced total panic. I still can't eat curry without feeling guilty. And I drink water almost exclusively.

25 Don't lie about how much you've eaten.

Many many people do this and I have to ask, what is the point? It's a waste of time. If the amount of weight you gained were directly related to how much you *thought* you ate, then, sure, this would be a sensible approach, but it's not. First of all, who cares? I'm a grown-up; I'm allowed to eat as much as I want. Wow, just *typing* that sentence seemed to do me a lot of good. I think I might try repeating it ten times: *I'm allowed to eat as much as I want. I'm allowed to eat as much as I want. I'm allowed to eat as much as I want. I'm allowed to eat as much as I want. I'm allowed to eat as much as I want. I'm allowed to eat as much as I want. I'm allowed to eat as much as I want. I'm allowed to eat as much as I want. I'm allowed to eat as much as I want. I'm allowed to eat as much as I want. I'm allowed to eat as much as I want. I'm allowed to eat as much as I want. I'm allowed to eat as much as I want. I'm allowed to eat as much as I want.*

All right, I guess that's fourteen, but it was making me feel so good, it was hard to stop at ten. Okay, so now I know I'm allowed to eat as much as I want and SO ARE YOU. You won't get thrown in jail, you won't get fired, you won't lose your children. Well, all right, if the truth be told, you very well might lose your husband or boyfriend, but as I hope I said earlier, if he doesn't make you feel safe, no loss.

Why Tell the Truth?

So why tell myself the truth of how much I eat? For one thing, if I lie about how much I've eaten, I'll then think it's okay to eat more. "Well, I've only had that one little breast of chicken . . ." I might say, when, in truth, I'd had two rolls while waiting for the chicken to arrive (and when it came, it was covered with butter sauce). And I had half my mother's ravioli. And a couple of bites of her crème caramel.

Also, it's a terrible idea to get in the habit of lying to yourself. I'm sure ALL of my therapists would agree. Because if I'm lying to myself about how much I eat—which once you think about it, is patently ridiculous—then *for sure* I am lying to myself about other things, too. And, when I tell myself something, I tend to believe it; I'm never clever enough to consider that I might be lying to myself. This is dangerous. You can just imagine. What if I lied to myself about my ability to operate heavy machinery? Or to keep state secrets?

And, even worse, lying to myself about how much I've eaten is fattening in another way.

How? Because lying makes me feel guilty. It induces a nagging feeling that something is wrong. And you know what? That nagging feeling can usually be alleviated by food. So all around, it's way better for me to just admit when I eat a lot. That doesn't mean I have to trumpet it to the world. It's not necessary to announce first thing when I meet someone "Hi, my name is Jane and I ate fifteen health food toffee bars today while lounging on the couch and reading Norah Lufts." No. But on the other hand, what do I have to gain by pretending that something is not true when it is? What I find is that if I just accept that I ate a lot on Wednesday and it's fine, I admit it and accept it, I have a much easier time not eating quite so much on Thursday.

26 Shop for clothes.

Shopping for clothes uses the same part of the brain as eating does. Research scientists have shown: it is not possible to think about food when you are shopping (unless you are wildly hungry or you try on enough clothes that look bad and you are sent into a depression).

Remember, it is completely possible to shop for clothes with NO intention of buying them or even trying them on. When I am too roundish to look good in most clothes (happened this very week, since, as I might've already told you, I am about one foot tall and have the shortest legs in the world, five extra pounds makes a department store dressing room a sure route to suicidal depression for me), I go shopping for clothes I will buy later BUT DON'T TRY THEM ON. I *imagine* that if I tried them on, I would look deeply sexy. (I can always convince myself that I will look voluptuous in an outfit as long as there is no evidence to the contrary.) But I do find that if I shop, even if I actually am hungry, the hunger goes completely away.

It took me a long time to learn this clothes shopping/food relationship because mostly I've been poor and, let's face it, there's only so much you can spend on food in one day and it's a lot less than you could theoretically spend on clothes. For example, I read recently that Cher spent $10,000 on one dress. No matter how piggish I was feeling, no matter how upscale the restaurants, it would not be possible for me to spend $10,000 on food in one day.

But what was I saying? Ah yes. How did I find out about this shopping thing? What transformative experience occurred? In my late thirties, I started dating an MTV director who was much younger than me. He was sexy, wildly funny and brilliantly talented. However, the relationship was not trouble-free. For one thing, he was quite interested in being popular with girls. He had spent a lifetime developing his pick-up ability only to have me come along and snatch him up just when he reached a tip-top pinnacle of skill and it grated on him not to get to use that super-power. Plus I was bossy and he was stubborn.

Now don't get me wrong, most of the time we got along wonderfully and had a great time but we did break up about every nine months or so. So one time when we were broken up—he was dating me and kind of trying to talk me into getting back together—I said, "Okay, I'll get back together with you, but you know what? You have a lot more money than me and whenever we break up, I wind up living in some rundown apartment with a graduate student roommate and a moldy shower, and that's not right. So yes, I'll get back together with you but only if you give me some money if we break up again."

So long story slightly shorter, about a year later, I found myself broken up with the MTV director boyfriend and with a lot of money. So every day I went shopping in Soho. I didn't spend the entire day shopping, just a couple of hours every morning. After just a few weeks of this I became quite a bit, greatly, remarkably thinner. The shopping had the same effect as eating. I was calmed and contented.

Of course, one might argue that it was how I looked in the clothes that made me eat less. (Like I read once that yoga makes you thin partially because you see how your stomach looks all squished up in front of your face.) But no, I know that's not true. For me, thinness always comes from happiness, never from shame.

27 Don't sit down to eat at a party thinking to be on a diet.

It's too damned difficult. Sometimes I'm at a wedding and they have great salmon and chinese pea pods and that's all I eat, but the much more likely scenario is that because I've been eating very little in order to look good for the wedding, I'm ravenous by the time I wake up that day. (By the way, did you know that men are made wildly romantic by weddings? It's true, so this is one of the TOP events you should diet for.) And I've usually had to dash around like a maniac getting ready and then expend enormous effort to get to the wedding, either running a mile across the L.A. Arboretum or parking on the far side of the field (well, okay, with some weddings you can just take a taxi to the door of the hotel and travel by elevator to the roof), or flying in from Heathrow and—now let me catch my breath—after killing myself to arrive, right at that moment the ceremony starts and then everyone stands around wondering where the reception is. Finally, *finally*, when I've waited in line for the buffet or for the waiters to get to my table which is inevitably the absolute last table they serve, I am definitely not going to delicately turn down boeuf en croute, NO, I AM GOING TO TRY NOT TO EMBARRASS MYSELF BY ASKING FOR TWO.

Remember that pain and torture are not good. Unless of course, you're in the mood for pain and torture. Then they're okay.

And besides, I have a hard time being a good guest if I am ravenous and tortured. It's important to be an amusing and accomplished guest. So I allow myself to eat freely.

Check This Out: Andy Warhol's Diet

This party business reminds me of Andy Warhol's diet because he had to eat out every night with a group. It was torment for him because he was naturally roundish and needed to be very very thin to fit in with his chosen group of New York glitterati (or maybe to sport that crazy wig). So, what he would do was go to a restau-

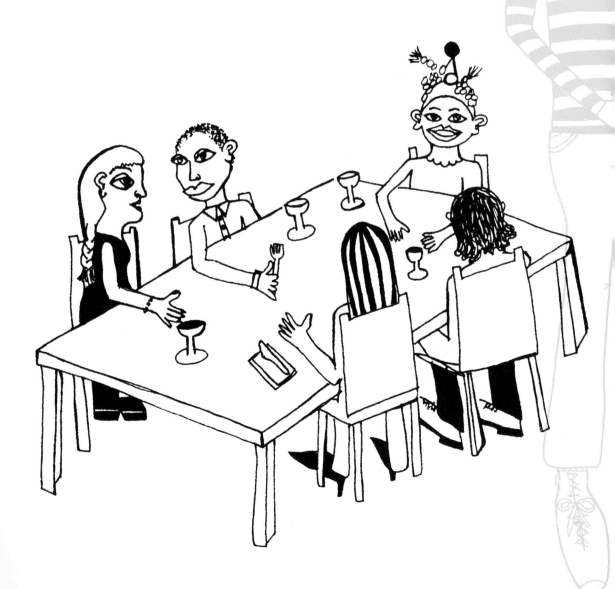

rant and order three dishes he didn't like, say, oysters, sweetmeats and menudo. He would be quite hungry and, unfortunately, sitting and watching other people eat always makes you feel like eating too, so he would say to himself "Maybe I'll like oysters now," and then he'd take a bite but no, they were still horrible. Then after a few minutes, he'd think "What about sweetmeats? Maybe they're not so bad." Again a bite. Yuck. Then he'd try the menudo.

By the time he'd done this a couple of times, he was full enough, the dinner was over and he'd survived only ingesting about 200 calories. Then he'd get his leftovers packed and give the box to a homeless person on the street.

Now of course this is not a terribly practical plan (and maybe not that nice to the homeless either), but I thought I'd mention it. What I do most of the time when eating out is: try to follow this rule: I have some non-fattening things first and then throw caution to the winds, imagining that caution will be returned by those very same winds to my doorstep early tomorrow morning or tomorrow afternoon at the latest.

28] Try not to obsess about food. (Yeah, like I'm even remotely capable of taking this advice.)

My ultimate goal is never to feel like there are things I want and cannot have. My immediate goal is to convince myself that while I can have any food I want, it just so happens that right this minute I want stir-fried green beans. (And, curiously, the more I have green beans, the more I do, indeed, want them.)

The problem with being on A DIET is that once I start deny-
ing myself something, I want it all the more. I might as well
just insist that I must be celibate. That would be a disaster of equal
proportions. You know what would happen.

Think of it like this: What if you decided you could never
go into your bedroom between seven and ten at night? Here's
what would happen: between seven and ten every night you would
desire nothing so much as to go into your bedroom. You would
long for the bedroom and when you forgot your longing for even
a second, you would find yourself thinking of a reason to go to
the bedroom and you'd get halfway there, then remember the
rule. You would reluctantly convince yourself not to go into your
bedroom. Mr. or Ms. Right could be in the living room whis-
pering the most amusing sweet nothings in your ear while gaz-
ing at you with obvious desire and admiration, but you would
still wish they would go away so you could concentrate more
on your bedroom.

Moral: the problem of denial is a toughie.

What Happened When The Very Thin Jenny Smith Went On a Diet

Jenny Smith (not her real name) was a girl who started board-
ing school with me in the early seventies. When she arrived at the
school she was 5'6" and weighed 85 pounds. After a few months,
she noticed that the rest of us were on a diet and she decided to
go on a diet, too. We were outraged because she was ALREADY
too thin so we reported her to the headmistress, indignantly insist-
ing that she be stopped. (I'm sure any normal person would have
been outraged by the rest of us being on a diet too; most of us
probably weighed around 115 lbs.) The headmistress talked to
Jenny, but what could she do? She couldn't watch Jenny every
second. So, Jenny desperately tried to eat very very little during
the next two weeks. What happened? At the end of the two weeks,
Jenny had gained 15 pounds. By concentrating on something that
had earlier come naturally to her, she achieved the exact opposite
result than what she desired.

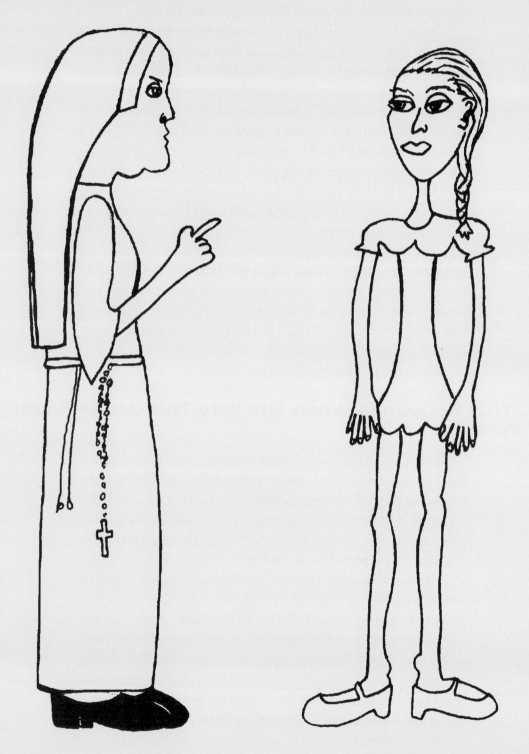

Eeks, Jenny had gained 15 pounds

The lesson is obvious! Ideally, no one should ever be on a diet! Your natural way of eating should be okay to keep your weight about the same, month after month. Every once in a while that has been true for me and I have been able to go happily along at a nice weight (112 is so lovely for me). Then I don't think about what I'm eating that day and I don't actually think that much about food. But in order for this to happen, conditions have to be pretty close to perfect.

Setting Up Perfect Conditions

What constitutes perfect life conditions for me might be different than perfect conditions for you.

For one thing, as I said before, I am driven completely crazy by being penniless. I go into a panic, my mind darting frantically around: How am I going to eat? Sure, I could go over to Mike and Sarah's house but what if they are having tuna noodle casserole? I know I'd eat a lot of it and be deeply sorry later. What if there's no money for food *tomorrow*? What if I never get to EAT AGAIN?!!

When that happens I have to eat A LOT.

Once, when I was living in Texas, my friend Lucy and I had only about $4, not enough money for food for the both of us, so I got the bright idea that we would go to a bar, order a beer and then wait for someone to pick us up and take us out to dinner. Well, we did meet these two really nice guys. In fact, as I remember, they might have made good boyfriends but I was concentrating way too hard on eating to pay attention to them even slightly. They asked if we wanted to go to their aunt's house out by the lake. I think Lucy made some small objection, but to me "House = Food," so I accepted with alacrity. When we got there I made a beeline for the refrigerator. "Anything to eat in here?" The guy who had decided I was his date, who also happened to be the one with the aunt, laughed nervously. "I don't know if you wanna eat just anything, but there's some birthday cake left over from Saturday." So, that's what I had, three-day-old white birthday cake.

That was bad.

More Perfect Conditions

I have to have a boyfriend who's nice to me. Particularly good is a boyfriend who will do whatever I want. Whenever that has happened I have lost weight without having to worry about it too much.

I went out with a guy once. Wonderful. Affectionate. Loving. Got me through the very tumultuous years of 19 to 23. He called me "my every waking thought." After the early good-behaviour phase of our relationship wore off, we'd go out and I would insist that we order three entrees. I would then eat all of mine, all of the second one and half of his. (He was pretty thin and didn't eat much.) In the car on the way home, I would lie on the front seat, unbutton my pants and groan about how full I was. Occasionally he would gently point out that perhaps I would be more comfortable if I ate only, say, two meals. After about six months with him, I started eating only one-and-a-half meals, then just my own, and then sometimes not even all of mine. Eventually, I ate only until I was full and I became quite thin. For once I was "getting enough" (love and affection) and I was safe.

Thirdly

I can't be working a terrible job. A terrible job is one where the boss is crazy, mean, immoral or stupid. I have at this point worked about 250 jobs, and I'd have to say that the bosses in about 240 of them were terrible. Working a bad job, I need padding, and I definitely acquire extra weight for protection. Now, as soon as I start getting fatter on a job – I quit.

And Fourth

I have to have a bathtub. When I live in a house with only a shower, I gain twenty pounds immediately. I need a full-length mirror . . . I need . . . But enough of the particulars. The principle is what's important. The point is that if I figure out what conditions are ideal for me and strive to create them, weight melts off. The obsession disappears. If I can feel that I am rich in every way, the weight problem takes care of itself.

Juice is a great invention. 29

Particularly vegetable juice. Carrot juice, beet juice, and especially green juice. Very few calories, good taste, fills you up. Contains lots of nutrients, fabulous for the appearance.[27] Also, on those occasions when I am desperately hungry but want my stomach to be full for only half an hour or so (dinner party coming up, going to yoga, about to go to sleep), juice is the perfect food.

A Beautiful Juice Story

My friend Roseanne was once quite lovely and the object of much male attention. (Both Prince Charles *and* Mick Jagger tried to pick her up—now *that's* something.) She lived in Houston and had a terrible boyfriend for ten years, then finally moved to Los Angeles to get away from him. Soon after she got there, she began working for *The Los Angeles Times* in the advertising department. Her boss agreed to move her into editorial as soon as there was an opening, but, because she was such a good worker, he secretly and repeatedly blocked any hope she had of getting transferred, even when editors asked for her specifically. During a fifteen-year period she became quite roundish, very roundish in fact.

Eventually she moved to Northern California, found a great house and began pursuing her dream of screenwriting. Weight began to peel off, but not quickly enough to suit her. Then, one day, she stumbled into Jamba Juice. She discovered that if, around ten a.m. every day, she bought a super-deluxe fresh-squeezed Berry Fulfilling (berry smoothie: raspberry juice blend, frozen strawberries, frozen raspberries, frozen blueberries, ice and something called "enlightened base," which she only knew was not as fattening as sherbet), she could nurse it all day long and then have a small dinner of mainly vegetables and go to bed totally satis-

27 Learn more about juice: Juicing For Life by Cherie Calbom and Maureen Keane.

fied. No suffering whatsoever, and she lost 100 pounds in slightly less than a year.

Small Discussion of Certain Juices Demonstrating the Quite Frightening Depth of My Obsession

This is a bit of an exception to the no-liquid-calories idea (see Hint #24, Don't Drink Anything With Calories) because, of course, juice has calories. Carrot juice, though, has very few calories, enough antioxidants to make an elephant's skin smooth, and is fantastically, massively, beautifully delicious.

I myself love wheatgrass juice, love the very *idea* of that many vitamins in a one-ounce drink. That tiny shot of wheatgrass takes care of practically all the nutrients you need for the day, maybe even the week. Many people think that wheatgrass juice tastes vile, but I come from a grass-eating background (As a small child I ate grass, paper and wool. I used to eat my school uniform and when I was in first grade, my mother had a bet with the next door neighbor as to whether I would chew through the straps by the end of the year (the straps held out, but of course I was very aware of the need to be careful)), so to me it's delicious. I believe everyone would come to love wheatgrass juice once they got used to it. If you've been eating a lot of bad things, like McDonald's hamburgers or croissants, wheatgrass may make you feel kind of nauseous. But this is easily fixed: simply avoid wheatgrass if you've been overly indulgent.

Another Useful Juice Suggestion

If I am driving and become incredibly hungry and the only place to stop is a little gas station convenience store, often the only good food is tomato juice. I allow myself to have two.[28] [29]

28 According to Max Gerson, whose specialty is curing diseases through a mainly juice diet and coffee enemas (NOTE: This diet is worth looking up and his book is fabulous although again, please remember, I am a total sucker for a miracle cure, but I do digress.), it's better to have a hydraulic press because centrifugal juicers destroy some of the good juice benefits. I am not yet able to afford this luxury but I'm eagerly looking forward to owning this strange-and-expensive-health-contraption in the not-too-distant future.

29 Read about it: A Cancer Therapy: Results of Fifty Cases and the Cure of Advanced Cancer by Max Gerson.

Be Patient With Juice

One more thing about juice: it's difficult to prepare and requires a lengthy ritual. Even if your role is simply to stand at the health food counter and watch the girl cut the fresh wheatgrass with special scissors and then jam it into the small hole of the cast iron grinder which ferociously squeezes the grass until it yields up liquid, or to stand patiently and watch her carefully pick out the carrots from one bin and beets from another (by law, apparently, kept as far as possible from the juicer), you still feel a part of an arcane ceremony. That's fine. Get into it. Obsessives like elaborate and complicated rituals.

It is best to eat fruit, by itself, first thing in the morning. 30

Evidently your liver likes that. It's easy to process, so the liver can continue the cleansing process it started the night before. It's good to take milk thistle extract for your liver, too. Your liver is really a miraculous organ, it can be deeply damaged and still grow back. [30]

This Is Totally Gross

Here's another really disgusting fact, though. My father told me this one day when I was about thirteen. We were standing on the lawn looking back at the house and he said, "You know those big stomachs that some men, well, mostly men, have called 'beer bellies'? In actual fact they *are* beer bellies. When someone drinks too much alcohol their liver can no longer filter the blood from their intestines and the serum leaks through into the abdominal cavity (which is supposed to be empty). This is a condition

[30] Read about your liver:
The Fat Flush Plan, by Ann Louise Gittelman

called 'acites' and when doctors drain the fluid they get as much
as nine or ten quarts of liquid."

I find this deeply disgusting. It's a bit like having sewage stored
in a bag inside you. An internal colostomy bag.

The Extreme Difficulty of Being Happy

One of the themes of this book is how to control the inevitable
damage that occurs when you succumb to excess.

It *is* possible to have a good life if you manage to do two things.
One is: contain the damage, which means, don't hurt yourself
worse than can be repaired and ALSO do the repair work as soon
as possible. The second thing is a thousand times more difficult
because most people *expect* everything to go wrong for them. The
expectation that everything will go wrong exists because, quite
simply, that *is* their experience. And it so often *is* their experience because that is what they expect. The self-fulfilling prophecy
in action.

Here is what you must do in order to have a good life: PRE-
PARE YOURSELF TO HANDLE THINGS GOING WELL.
Happiness is difficult to handle. You must make yourself into a
person who is comfortable being happy.

Here's how I learned this: Years ago, before I had ever met a
celebrity or come into contact with any of my heroes, I read
one day in the paper that Jules Feiffer was going to be signing
books at a book store near my house on a Saturday in about a
month. Now, he may not be a big deal to you, but Jules Feiffer,[31]
political cartoonist, storyteller and essay writer, is someone I hold
in high regard. He is silly and funny while never betraying the
seriousness of his subject matter. So when I saw that he'd be making an appearance, I thought, "Hey, I can go see him," but immediately afterward thought, "Nah, it won't happen. I'll never remember or I'll have to work. Something will prevent me so there's no
use even trying to remember the date." Then I put the matter out
of my mind.

Well, about a month later, I was walking down the street, no-

31 All the Jules Feiffer books are good. Don't look for an instant pay off, though. Try Munro,
Tantrum, and By the Side of the Road. www.julesfeiffer.com.

thing much to do, wondering how to waste several hours before it was time to go to work. Then I remembered: Jules Feiffer was at the bookstore that very day! "But where is the store?" I wondered. Why, it was very near where I was! Then I thought, "Well, I had wanted to take him one of my books of cartoons but I don't have one with me." Disappointed for a moment, I suddenly realized that I did have one at the restaurant where I worked, only a few blocks away!

So I got my book and went to the bookstore. I bought a book from Jules Feiffer and somehow managed to screw up the courage to give him one of mine, talked to him for a few seconds, then, completely overwhelmed, rushed out of there and took a cab to work.

As I was being driven down the street, I began experiencing the most uncomfortable feeling and wished I could stop it. It felt like someone had pumped air between the skin and the bone of my skull. "What is this unfamiliar feeling?" I thought. I finally got it: this is happiness. On the heels of that realization came a second one: *most people* are uncomfortable with happiness simply because it is unfamiliar to them. They would rather have a boss who was mean to them and a wife who burned the dinner because that was what they were COMFORTABLE with. That is what they were used to. And if I wanted to be able to experience *more* happiness, I was going to have to remember to "force" myself to be comfortable with it whenever it occurred until the comfort became automatic.

People are comfortable with what they know. What they don't know—even if it's good—can be unpleasant at first. In order to be happy, it's necessary to learn to tolerate being uncomfortable for a bit. That goes for being thin, too.

Make an attempt to chew each bite fifty times. 31

This is something I have never been able to do. In a way, it's surprising since part of the reason I like to eat is that I love to chew (see Hint #22). You would think that I'd like to chew each bite a million times but, paradoxically, I don't. I always try to remember to chew more and lately I've been making a truly concerted effort because I read a book about how difficult it is to digest food that has not been chewed enough.[32] Strangely, I always seem to forget. It's as if my specific number of chews-per-mouthful were set when I was a kid and now anything else feels unnatural. I hold out hope that I can retrain myself. After all, isn't that what a lot of these hints are about?

32 Having a slow metabolism is not completely bad.

For years, the bane of my existence as a roundish person was that my metabolism moves more slowly than the rate at which sedimentary rock accumulates. I can gain weight eating one celery stick a day.

And what's worse? The new news that when you go on a diet, your body thinks it might starve before some intrepid hunter can locate new meat, so it slows itself down even MORE so that now I can gain weight on *half* a stick of celery.

But, as I keep telling you, start to look at things in a different way. If your metabolism is slow, rejoice! Rejoice because this cloud has a very beautiful silver lining. If your metabolism is slow, you don't process food so quickly but, it also means *your entire body is revving at a slower rate,* so it's getting a lot less wear. Have

32 Read about chewing:
Mayo Clinic on Digestive Health.

you noticed that chubby women look much younger? That is not just because the fat has plumped out their wrinkles. They *are* younger. Naturally, the trick is to stay thin while having a slow metabolism, but if you can pull it off, you have been handed a golden ticket in the contest of youthfulness.

A Really Great Slow Metabolism Story

Once upon a time, there was a French family who lived in the Loire Valley. The father's uncle lived with them. At first the uncle helped around the house and in the garden, but as the years went by he did less and less. Finally it seemed he could do no more than get out of bed and move, with excruciating slowness, to sit in a chair, motionless and silent. When night fell, he moved, again very slug-gishly, back to bed. When the family realized the uncle might not recover from his tremendous deceleration, they called in doctors from near and far to find out what was wrong. No one could figure it out. Then one day a doctor came and proclaimed that there was nothing wrong with Uncle Pierre but an incredibly slow metabolism.

"Voila!" the French family exclaimed in their expressive French way and immediately administered medication to speed up his metabolism. Three months later Pierre died.

When an autopsy was performed, it turned out that the uncle had had liver cancer but because of his slow metabolism, it was growing at such a snail's pace that he probably would have lived for another twenty years had the medication not been adminis-tered to speed him back up to normal.

Now if you think about it, this story is not that sad because the uncle was already old and really, is it better to live for twenty years merely to sit in a chair all day? But surely you recognize the implications for your own, roundish self: slower metabolism means slower aging, slower wearing down of all body parts, longer life.[33]

And in some macro-ecological way, isn't it far better to use less of the world's resources to run the single organism that is you? If you are a slow metabolizer, give yourself a hearty pat on the back for your service to worldkind.

33 Read this: The Nutrition Solution: A Guide To Your Metabolic Type by Harold Kristal.

33 There is a size that my body wants to be.

If I kill myself to change this I might be making a terrible mistake.

My body has a natural size and being another size can involve an enormous struggle for very little upside. This doesn't mean my body's natural size is 200 pounds and there's nothing I can do about it. No. However, if I normally weigh 120, then that weight is very easy for me to maintain and I can pretty much eat what I want. But to be 115 or (whew!) 112, I have to work really really hard and if I turn my back for a second, my body quickly scarfs up a bunch of pancakes and goes back to 120. 120 feels good to it. It loves 120.

Actually, I'm pretty much happy with my natural size but I do have this one dress that only looks good if I weigh less. There's a small pocket of fat right on my hips and another one in the saddlebag, upper thigh area. No amount of exercise makes these problem areas go away, they only disappear on the rare occasions when I'm super-skinny.

Theoretically I could have liposuction and perhaps if I become rich one day I will, but liposuction is a lot like plastic surgery: you have to be careful. I knew a woman, quite rich, quite beautiful in a swingy-hair, freckle-faced way who I'm pretty sure had liposuction and, I think, breast implants. She wound up looking eerily strange. Her butt was round in the back, but kind of flat on the sides and her legs were like sticks. Her breasts, however, were quite large and so her proportions were odd to the point of deformity.

A Scary But Quite Interesting Story

In July of 1999, I went to a writing conference in Belize at the resort of a famous director (who shall remain unnamed). While there I contracted a very virulent form of parasites called entaemoeba histolytica which lives in your body and over time attempts to take over completely. It took about six months before I figured out what was going on. There were many odd things that started happening, most of which I won't go into right now, except to tell you the oddest, which was that I was getting bikini waxes at the time and at some point in September, about two months into the ordeal, my pubic hair no longer grew back. Convenient? Yes. A help to my budget? Definitely. But, as you might imagine, a bit disturbing, too. I mean, what kind of doctor do you see for that condition?

Then, in September, another curious thing started to happen. No matter how much I ate, I always lost weight. I was delirious with happiness. I thought, "Finally, God has given me the body I was meant to have all along." I ate my normal amount and I just kept getting thinner and thinner. And thinner. Even more delightfully, this all happened when I had a chunk of money (from breaking up with the MTV guy) and so I was able to go shopping for designer clothes and they did look completely spectacular.[34]

Unfortunately, the disease progressed to the point where I became a bit worried about how thin I had gotten (what a switch!) and just about that exact time, I got two pains in the lowest part of my stomach, just inside my hip bones. As it turned out, another girl had also contracted the disease (same resort, same consequence) but her symptoms appeared about a week ahead of mine. Luckily for me, she'd just graduated top of her class from Princeton and so had already researched and gotten all the best doctors.

Curing the disease was quite difficult and required many series of antibiotics, followed by a lot of lying in bed and eating nothing but brown rice and vegetables. Five *months* of eating brown rice and cooked vegetables.

Basically you have to use every method possible to kill off what are small, extremely dangerous organisms trying to colonize your

34 Okay, just got back from Camp Full Disclosure. I know that earlier I said it was the shopping itself that made me thinner and now here I claim strange tropical disease. It was the latter but I swear, the shopping as a diet strategy helped, too.

body and claim it as their own. I imagined them a guerrilla army living in the country of my body. They got the food supplies first, but I determined what food we ate. Food that they didn't like was left for me. (Mainly cooked vegetables, rice and pumpkin seeds.) Also, their main force was wiped out with the antibiotics, but that still left the guerrilla outposts stationed in the hills and every one of them had to be killed or they could breed and come back.

So the total miracle of weight loss that I thought was happening turned out to be naught but a strange tropical disease. (This was the exception to: There Is A Size That My Body Wants to Be. And let me tell you, this opposite was not good.)

But all that being said, the experience of losing weight so easily also taught me that anything is possible.

Anything Is Possible

Last year I went to my boyfriend's house for Christmas and New Year's. On Christmas Eve his brother and I were sitting at a long wooden table in his parent's kitchen (which is a converted barn) looking at some photographs. It just so happened that two pictures of his father were in close proximity to each other. One of the photos was only a few weeks old while the other had been taken about three years earlier, just before he had been diagnosed with leukemia, the slow-acting kind that strikes mainly older men and kills them in fifteen to twenty years. At the time his father contracted it, he was seventy. He underwent a rather rigorous regimen of chemotherapy which left him weak and vulnerable for a couple of years to every small germ that wandered by. In the long run, he was cured.

But at the time I was looking at these pictures, that entire struggle was in the past; it was the pictures themselves that were interesting. In the older photo, he was very thin, his hair was greyish-white and he looked his age, which was strange to see because my boyfriend's father usually looked much much younger. But by the time of the recent photos, he had gained back his bulk, looked young again and most amazingly, *his hair had turned back to dark red.* I was completely amazed.

As it happens, his father was actually sitting right across from me at the table, and I looked up from the photographs to see that, sure enough, he did not have one grey hair on his head.

My immediate thought was: if this guy's hair could turn back to dark red at the age of 72, anything is possible. [35]

Of course, these examples—that maybe miracles do happen and hair and bodies can miraculously change—illustrate the exact opposite of what I'm trying to say, which is *do not* long for a different body than you have. Sure, I have spent a LOT of time imagining what my life would have been like if I had my mind inside Elle McPherson's body, but that's ridiculous. I have to remind myself almost every day that my mind (of which I am quite fond and wouldn't trade for all the oil in Byelorussia) only developed because it was attached onto a body which, although perfectly serviceable, wasn't going to get me elected prom queen. [36]

And although having Karen Elson's shape would have probably made absolutely everything I've ever tried to do immensely easier in the long run, I might not have turned out funny. And that would just be hell. The very idea of trying to confront the vicissitudes of everyday life without a sense of humor makes me shudder.

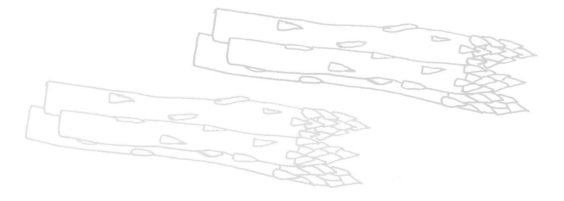

[35] Some time later, I happened to come across an article in *The Guardian* which reported on a medicine for leukemia that turns white hair back to its original color. Hmm. Perhaps he took this medicine. Even if he did, that would not make the hair color change any less miraculous as far as I'm concerned.

[36] Okay, yes. I *was* prom queen. But I was *not* elected. I invented the office and appointed myself. How that happened is a long story that mainly involves the fact that my younger brother John was so cool, I was allowed to get away with this simply by being his relative, a fact I was well aware of when I dreamed the scheme up.

34. For two weeks each month my body likes to be fatter and will insist I eat more.

This would be the two weeks before my period. You cannot imagine how many times I have been deeply distressed that there just seemed no way for me to keep from eating a lot during these pre-period periods. **36.2**

The Other Two Weeks

Okay, so after I've been furiously sinking my teeth into every piece of fried chicken and ginger cookie in a five-mile radius for about four days, I remember that in the two weeks before my period my body likes to be a bit fatter, uh, rounder. Then, once my period begins, I have absolutely no trouble with a 400-calorie a day diet (have you noticed any tendency on my part to exaggerate?) and the weight just melts right off. Then two weeks later, I'm berating myself for my lack of control again.

The whole thing is totally ridiculous. No one notices but me. Am I afraid that my friends will refuse to hang out with me? "Oh my God, I can't be her friend anymore, she's too fat."

Or will my boyfriend, who's madly in love, break up with me? "I'm sorry. I love you, but those five pounds you've put on in the

36.2 I'll pause here and say that I hope men who are reading this book do not feel alienated. I think men have cycles too, but since they are not so clearly demarcated, men have a harder time noticing them. I think, and this is totally theory, but I think that if men paid closer attention and figured out their cycles, it would make the efficient running of their bodies easier. But that's just me. Who knows? Maybe they don't want to know their cycles. Maybe the best bet is leaving well enough alone.

last week makes it a 'no go'." I'd be there on my knees, crying, begging him to wait another ten days when I would be thin again. "I promise I will, I promise," I'd sob. I mean, maybe if I gained twenty pounds he would leave me, but *five?*

The best thing to do is to try to just relax and accept this. No sense becoming suicidal every month over something you can't do anything about anyway. Suicidal impulses are better saved for real horrors like making a mistake on the job or missing an important phone call.

This doesn't mean *I* can relax. I still have to apply all my eating hints and struggle as hard as I can during this monthly battle. Obviously, I can't just eat my head off for two weeks and expect to stay svelte. But I do try to remind myself that when I lose the struggle (more often than not), it's not from lack of willpower. There are some battles that simply cannot be won. **37**

My theory is to try as hard as you can. Trying works, in my opinion; you do reap rewards.

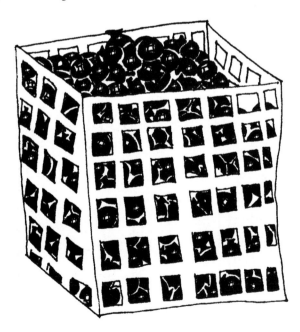

---

37 I'm pretty sure there is a great quote from The Art of War that could be used here about how you have to lose some battles to win the war, but never having read that book even during its heyday as Mike Ovitz's Bible, none come to mind.

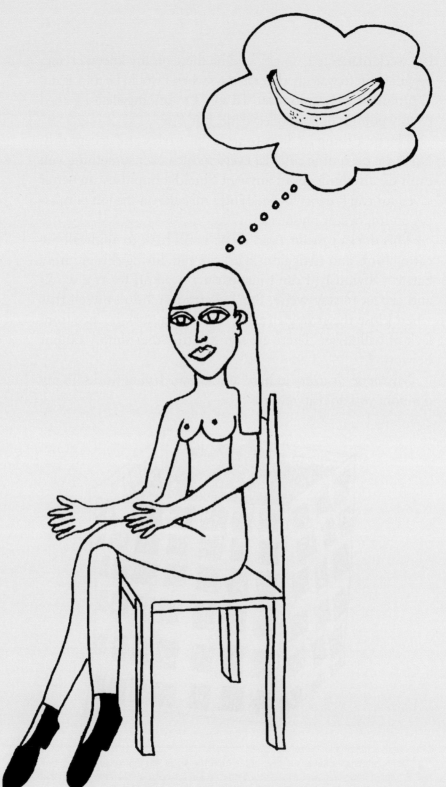

If a food pops into your mind, go get it. Right away.

When I get a craving, particularly for a food considered healthy, I pay attention.

35

My body tells me very precisely what it needs if I just listen. Sometimes an actual picture of the food will appear in my mind. And I always try to have these foods as soon as possible, never mind what kind of eating plan I had in mind for that day.

Usually it will be something like a banana or a hamburger. (But I do try to remind myself: there's no need to eat the bun with the hamburger.)

Never never ever ever ever weigh yourself.

36

Some people love to weigh themselves. (Hey, some people work for a tyrant for years, some people are low-level Mafia henchmen, and some people walk around with blackened and missing teeth. It takes all kinds.) For me, getting on a scale every morning is a terrible mistake because it makes me depressed. And then in order to feel better I would have to eat two breakfasts. Which would be a bad idea.

C A S E   H I S T O R Y   N O . 1 7

Sam Freaks Out

Sam was a roundish fellow who lived in Munich. An American working for a German company, he was often on the road, meeting with his salesmen, and would usually eat whatever was available. This was okay with him, but because he really liked food, when he came home and was able to relax, he tried to have *great* meals. Three-cheese lasagna or green chili stew with tortillas, a delicious pot roast and occasionally, knockwurst. He didn't exactly overeat, it was just that he broke every rule in this book. Also, he loved wine. [38] He was a connoisseur. There was nothing he liked better than sharing a bottle with his lovely wife after the children were in bed, or having some friends over on a Saturday afternoon for a wine tasting.

The bad food habits and the wine had added a few pounds, he didn't know how many, but he did know that it was more than he used to carry when he was young. He didn't really mind – after all, he was a businessman and the added heft made him look serious. Or at least that's what he told himself when it even crossed his mind, which happened about twice a year. He might have gone on quite happily like this for the rest of his life but one day a cataclysmic event took place. He was at The American Club for a game of tennis and he happened to glance over and notice that they had a doctor's scale in the men's dressing room. After he finished tying up his shoes, he went over and stood on the scale.

TWO HUNDRED AND THIRTY POUNDS! He was aghast. He had gained thirty pounds since he last weighed himself. He stayed calm (that was his nature), giving no outward indication that he had totally freaked, but by the time he was halfway through the match, he had decided something must be done.

Sam went right out and bought a home scale and determined to weigh himself every day. All of a sudden, his weight

---

38 Have I said anything about alcohol? Not really. Alcohol is pretty fattening unless you give up on food completely. Which is a bad Idea. If you are a man and drink beer everyday, give it up for a a week and see what happens. You won't believe it.

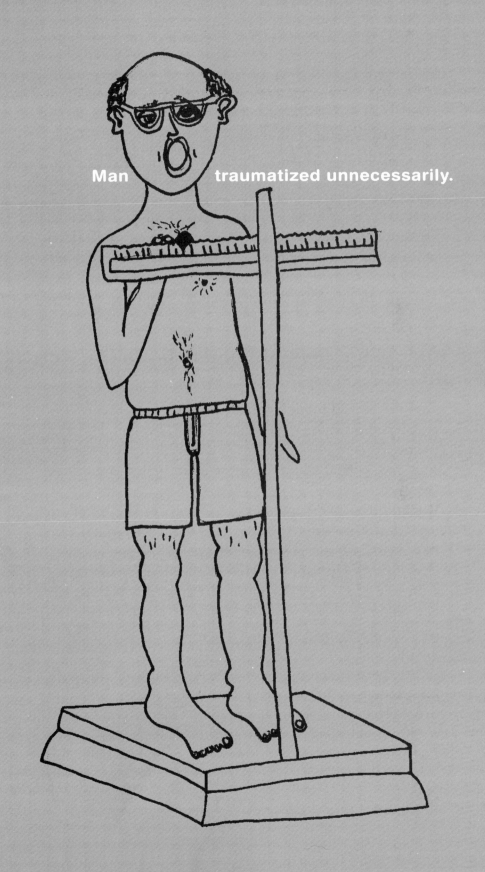

became a focus—the main focus, in fact—of his attention. As he would reach for a second sandwich he would tell himself that he wasn't allowed. Then a few hours later, in the middle of the afternoon, he'd send his secretary for a couple of candy bars to "perk himself up." His gourmet meals got just a little bit bigger. Every day he weighed himself. He never lost weight. On the contrary, by the end of the first week, he'd gained two pounds! He went into a depression. He was always hungry. After a month he was no longer thirty pounds heavier than he had been, he was FORTY POUNDS heavier!

Here's the lesson: do *not* weigh yourself, it will merely depress you.[39]

The Ridiculousness of Focussing on An Actual Weight

What do you think you *should* weigh? 105 pounds? 110 pounds? You're wrong. Unless you are under five foot three, that is too little. It's the weight of an anorexic. When you get on the scale and see that you do not weigh that much you will be depressed.

But. If you *don't* get on the scale, what's to keep you from believing you weigh 115 pounds? Nothing. Then you lose a little weight, now you believe you only weigh 110 pounds. Who cares if you really went from 125 to 120? Losing weight is so great, you'll feel like losing more. (Hmmm, this may actually be a case in which you *should* lie to yourself. Ideally you shouldn't care what weight you are, but I find I do. So yes, in this instance, I lie.)

If you're happy, you'll lose weight; if you are depressed you'll gain it. It's that simple – have your family tell you how thin you look all the time. It doesn't matter if they don't sound truthful, your subconscious will still believe them. Try it. If someone says, "Oh my god, you've lost so much weight. You look wonderful!" What do you feel like doing? Cheering. On

39 Oh, and don't worry about Sam. Eventually he found out about food combining and, like George, lived happily ever after.

the other hand if they say, "Geez, you've gotten a little chunky. Spending a lot of time in front of the TV?" What happens then? You go right out and buy some potato chips.

All right then. Why buy a machine that insults you first thing every morning? Why? So you can hate yourself?

If you have a scale, throw it out. Now.

Bouillon. 37

Bouillon (and I'm including miso here) is a miracle food: good for you, hydrates you and fills you up at the same time. In fact, it's the only kind of water that makes me feel full for more than half an hour. I could, theoretically, get through an entire day on nothing but four cups of bouillon and then the next day probably be half my size. My body would lose some extra weight just out of respect for the fact that in disciplining myself, I had gone to such an admirable extreme.

But now I'm going too far. The urge to drink bouillon only happens every now and again, but when it occurs, bouillon is exactly right and when those moments happen, I rejoice. (I mean, get out your surfboard and RIDE.) Like, let's say there's a day when I am totally getting high on how strict I am being with myself (let's call this phenomenon 'Anorexic for a Day' and really, I never allow it to last longer than 24 hours) and I find I'm hungry just before I go to bed. Bouillon. And I'm sure you can imagine how smug I feel, snuggled under a comforter drifting off to sleep with a GREAT day of dieting under my belt.

Always keep some bouillon around the house. Just in case.

Oh, and by the way, other soup is good, too. It's non-fattening (well, all the sorts without cream are), nutritious and delicious. And actually, other soup might be even better than bouillon. Sometimes I eat basically just soup for several days. Usually in the winter. It's a pretty good diet technique.

38 When driving across the country, go to the grocery store.

Grocery stores are usually pretty easy to find (it will come as no surprise that many people (not just you and me) are concerned with food), which means that just about anyone you ask can give you directions. There, you'll find instantly accessible food. You can get cabbage, whose leaves make a very tasty little snack (particularly if you like spicy, because often they're kind of spicy), or pears, plums, melon, even popcorn already popped.

Here let me pause and say that the English and the French don't seem to have caught on to pre-packaged, already-popped popcorn yet, but I'm sure they are just thinking it over before jumping enthusiastically onto that bandwagon and when they do, they will wonder why they ever hesitated. Because popcorn is great.[40]

More Good Foods Instantly Available At Any Grocery, Anywhere

Hearts of palm, crackers, red peppers and applesauce.

There are many many delicious and non-fattening foods in a grocery store, all patiently waiting on the shelves for you.

I drove across the country with Mike McQueen a couple of times. Hmm, that's a little misleading: actually, *he* drove and I sat in the passenger seat and told stories. I didn't get my driver's license until I was thirty-one years old. Too scared. We frequently stopped at grocery stores. I liked it because it's definitely not a tourist activity. You get a feel for the actual town. When you're at the grocery store in Little Rock, Arkansas, for example, you know pretty much

[40] Despite what I said in my earlier footnote. See, just like the warning warned you: contradictions.

for sure that all the other people in the store actually *live* in Little Rock.

And don't forget the grocery store when it comes to any other kind of travel. You can go to the grocery store before a plane or train or bus ride. It's slightly more of a pain, because fruits and vegetables are heavy. (In fact, really the worst part about fruit is that it's heavy and the two worst parts about vegetables is that they are heavy and they require so much preparation. Particularly washing. And some vegetables need a *lot* of washing, like spinach. The carrying around you can deal with because carrying heavy objects is quite good for you, particularly if you are a girl. But washing and cutting are really not that much fun. Though, I suppose, it might be possible to develop a love of these activities, much like developing a love of being hungry.)

Carrying Things

While I'm (subtextually) on the subject of osteoporosis, I really should stress the point again (see Hint #6 Exercise is King) that carrying things is good for you. No, let me commit myself—it's *essential.* You know how you always hear about old women falling down and breaking their hip? Sometimes it's the reverse: their hip has broken and *that* causes them to fall. Do you want bones that fragile? No you don't.

The answer: weight-bearing exercise. In fact, I think it would be perfect for rock stars to use menopausal women as roadies. It's a job with bad pay, horrible hours (older people really do need less sleep) and not really that much glory, but for menopausal women it would have the extra, added benefit of all that lifting and carrying. And I'm pretty sure everyone would get in a lot less trouble.

One Stone, Many Birds. Or: Think Big

I like things to have more than one benefit. I like to kill two birds with one stone, and even more than that I like to kill ten birds with one stone. (In actual fact, I don't like to kill *any* birds, but you get my point.) Which means: carry those fruits and vegetables gratefully and happily.

39 Always have some food with you.

Oh my heavenly days, I can't believe I almost forgot this. One of the big big problems with eating well is that when I am hungry, I AM HUNGRY! I must eat RIGHT AWAY. As you can imagine, this can be a bit of a problem if, for example, I am in the middle of a delicate business negotiation or driving down the freeway at seventy miles an hour or just riding down the escalator of the London Underground. But, I have solved this problem. I am always prepared. I never leave home without food. An apple, a green pepper—my friend Suzanne likes raisins and nuts (slightly too fattening for me)—a cucumber (which has the additional amusement factor of how you look walking down the street eating a raw cuke)—a banana.

But this is très importante. Because if I don't have food with me, I find myself turning into a lunatic, who'll eat anything, INCLUDING, BUT NOT LIMITED TO, THE VERY EVIL FOOD, **FRENCH FRIES**, to stave off a complete emotional collapse.

I kid you not.

40 Candy is fattening and bad for everyone, including small children and very thin people.

Same goes for cakes and cookies. Just because the package says "fat free," so what? There's no fat because *sugar is not fat* and it's all sugar. I mean, suppose you were on a plane and it crashed in an African jungle and everyone else was killed, and the next morning you woke up in some mangled piece of twisted metal that was once a plane part (inadequately warmed by airline blankets) and you saw a sign that read, 'Polar Bear Free Area'? Would that make you feel safe? This is exactly like thinking that a candy bar is good for you because it doesn't contain fat.

Sugar is terrible for you.[41] It is bad for you like heroin is bad for you or crack cocaine is bad for you. It is a highly addictive substance, maybe more addictive than any other substance on the face of the earth. Proof? Look at how many people choose it as their favorite drug. I've given up many drugs in my life—alcohol, nicotine (twice), coffee (twice), pot and sugar—and I will tell you that not only was sugar the hardest to give up by far, but it also took me twice as long, during which time I thought of little else. Two years.

Rebecca and I Bond Over Our Common Addiction

I met my friend Rebecca at a posh dinner party in the loft of a magazine editor on Mott Street in downtown New York. When dessert came she overheard me refusing the chocolate gateau because I don't eat sugar. (Incidentally, this was not too much of a problem for me since I don't really like to eat at parties – when I'm eating I prefer not to be distracted by people talking. One of my great regrets is that I have never gotten the chance to truly enjoy hors d'oeuvres because they are only served at cocktail parties.

Anyway, when Rebecca overheard me say I didn't eat sugar, she told me she didn't either. Usually the first question out of someone's mouth at moments like this is "Diabetic?" but neither of us assumed that of the other. She told me her sugar story.

Rebecca had been working part-time for a lawyer in the old Newsweek Building on Fiftieth and Madison and one day in the

41 Read: <u>Sugar Blues</u> by William Duffy.
(One of Gloria Swanson's favorite books).

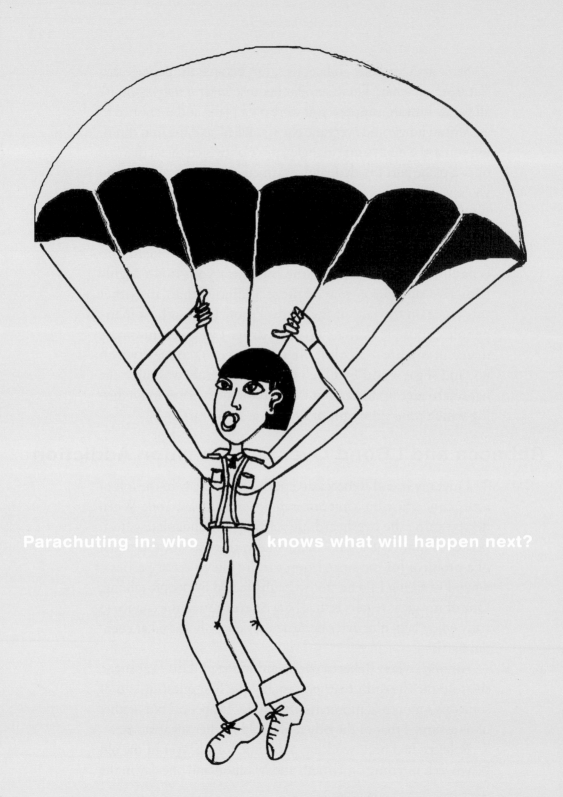

Parachuting in: who knows what will happen next?

elevator a stockbroker happened to offer her another part-time job in the same building as his assistant. She was barely making ends meet so she eagerly accepted. (Rebecca is a tall girl with masses of kinky curly dark brown hair, which tumbles in an unruly fashion down her back, despite her attempts to restrain it.)

Her workday went like this: 7 in the morning until 11 in the morning with the stockbroker, then the elevator up to the 41st floor from 11 to 3 with the lawyer, back down to the stockbroker from 3 to 7 pm. Both of the guys were busy enough to need full-time secretaries but they were getting a tremendous bargain in Rebecca and they knew it. In return, she was getting paid pretty well. It was, however, stressful.

After a few months, Rebecca had developed a routine. She tended to eat an entire box of cookies or six candy bars right about five o'clock at night which would render her passive and complacent enough to work all night long. One day she noticed that if she didn't get a sugar fix, she would turn into a raving maniac, barely restraining herself from yelling, "Get me the hell out of here," right around 5:30. She eventually realized that she was tolerating her very stressful work situation by getting high on sugar, using it as a drug. As soon as this thought occurred to her, she determined that when she left those jobs, she would kick the habit.

Getting off sugar was so difficult for her that whenever she sees a mother handing her child a candy bar or cupcake, in her mind's eye she sees, instead of the candy or cupcake, one of those small airplane bottles of booze because she deeply believes the two drugs are about equally dangerous.

Try quitting. You'll see how hard it is. Go ahead. I challenge you. When you find out how difficult it is, consider why.

Beautiful Beautiful Health Food Candy

I still eat health food candy, sweetened most preferably with rice syrup, bran malt, maple syrup or grape juice. Every once in a great while I eat food sweetened with honey or molasses. To be honest with you, health food candy is not that good for you either and one of these days I hope to give it up, too. But I do find a difference. For one thing, I don't *want* to eat two boxes of health food cookies; I can actually be happy with three single cookies. Also, I don't have the sudden high and then the intense drop that regular sugar gives, so it seems my body actually does process these types of sugar more slowly. More like a complex carbohydrate.

But there is a debate about whether health food candy (which is my generic term for health food sweets) is any different from regular candy, cookies or cakes.

About four years ago when I was living in New York City, my brother, who was living in Rye (a forty-minute train ride away), lost his nanny. The replacement couldn't start for a month so he and his wife asked me to be the interim nanny.

(By now you must be wondering what kind of job this crazy woman has that permits her to dash about everywhere and change her job every second. I'll tell you: Writer. And while I'm busily telling you how to live your life, I'll say right now: **Do not be a writer.** There is no money in writing. If you want to have even a modicum of financial security, do almost anything else.)

I loved the idea of nannying because I'm quite fond of their three children: Darst, the intellectual hellion; Caroline, who could spot fake Prada by the age of three (and with a mother who is SO not that); and Emily, who is quietly figuring things out for herself. So on a cold winter's day, I took the train up to their house and began working, doing all the things that nannies do.

Except one. I did not dispense sugar of any kind. I have told all my nieces and nephews that there is no way I will let them have sugar. I'm lenient in every other way, but they'll have to get their sugar from some other pusher. So I brought a supply of health food candy with me. On this particular day, it happened to be Sunspire chocolate pecan turtles, which are very delicious. Even people who sneer openly at health food nuts such as myself admit these candies are great. After lunch, when Darst asked for dessert, I delivered my "I'm not a pusher" spiel and gave him one of my candies. He took a bite. "Hey that's good," he said. He ate two more bites and then put down the candy, half-eaten, and ran off to play. And, for a change, committed no infractions of any rules that entire afternoon.

That was when I knew that health food candy was different not only for me, but for other people too.

Sugar is not beneficial for you. Let me repeat. It is cocaine, it is heroin, it is oxycontin. And one more thing (I realize I'm a bit hysterical on this subject. Maybe sugar isn't as bad for you as it is for me. You decide.): DON'T HAVE SUGAR FOR BREAKFAST.[42] Eat something else first, I beg you. Even a banana. Muffins, for example, are a terrible, terrible, terrible idea.

Yogurt is fattening. 41

Very fattening. Even plain yogurt. I like yogurt and, of course, now that I know it is a very fattening food, I love it even more, so what I do is have it when I go off my diet (and let me also say here that yogurt with flavoring is *abominable* food combining. The worst: sugar and protein) But. Big but: yogurt has lactobacillus acidophilus which is very beneficial if you have just taken antibiotics for some reason (which I hope was a good reason; antibiotics are not for casual use). So it's your call. Yogurt for healing, yogurt for fun, but definitely never yogurt for weight loss.

And I hope that was even slightly comprehensible. (At this point, in real life, if I were talking to you, I would wave my arms around in a haphazard fashion, as if to indicate that I am helpless to control my own brain.)

Keep away from salt. 42

Salt is another thing to stay away from, like cream and bread. It is quite delicious, but the curious thing about salt is that if you don't have any for three weeks you notice that your food tastes

---

42 Except the natural sugar in fruit. Fruit sugar is okay.

better without it. The taste of salt hides the other tastes. While conventional medicine holds that people with low blood pressure can eat all the salt they like, you have to watch out: some low blood pressure people turn into high blood pressure people.

When I first tried to give up salt, I thought I would die. I was living in New Mexico, working at the Albuquerque Country Club and, all of a sudden, food was tasteless. Life was no longer worth living. I got fat because I kept sampling more and more food, thinking "Maybe *this* chicken enchilada will have flavor. What about *those* tamales?" But then, slowly, it got better and all the flavor came back and, wow, I found I loved my food without salt even more.

Oh, and did I mention water retention? I'm not kidding when I say that giving up salt is one of the things which I believe made me slightly thinner permanently.

43 Fat, on the other hand, is not all bad.

French fries are bad. Very bad. It is true that French fries taste good. Sometimes I eat them even though the evidence now indicates that you might as well smoke an entire pack of cigarettes in terms of cancer-causing propensity, but you know, sometimes a French fry is so darned delicious, it's simply worth the risk. [43] [44]

But other fat-filled stuff is good for you: avocados, olive oil, tahini, flax seed. (Okay, this last is not in the category of "delicious food," but I do eat the seeds sometimes if I'm wanting to chew and don't care so much about flavor. The seeds kind of foam and swell up in your mouth in an interesting way).

43 Read <u>Fast Food Nation</u> by Eric Schlosser.

44 When British newspapers reported that French fries are cancer-causing, the experts said they were just considering the evidence that all carbohydrates are cancer-causing if fried or baked. I thought, "They're going to have to retract that. What would happen to the bread industry?" Sure enough, the statement was retracted, correctly or not, who knows? But I do have to say I now eat a lot fewer French fries and a lot more oatmeal.

You need oil to keep your insides greased. Your joints need oil and your skin needs oil, too. I can tell when someone eats too little oil; they start to look all cracked and dry like an old car seat.

A Radical Political Opinion

Let me draw your attention once again to women who are always on a diet.

Don't read any further if you're not interested in feminist politics.

It did occur to me once that dieting is the most brilliant strategy ever created in the history of humanity for one segment of the species to oppress another segment. How deeply convenient for men that women are always on a diet. And I don't think there had to be some kind of official committee meeting to come up with the plan of making women obsessed with their weight. Just like white men didn't have to have a *meeting* to decide to oppress black men. They do it naturally because they fear that black men's penises are bigger.

But think about it. What would you do if you had an enemy who you wanted to SLEEP beside you. What could be more brilliant than to convince them to weaken themselves? And the smarter and more driven they are, the more efficient they are at starving. And then, once they have starved themselves, not only are they always weak, but a huge portion of their brain cannot be concerned with political strategy because it is far too busy with thoughts like 'Get More Food' or 'I Hate Myself for Eating.' And how amazingly clever is the technique of holding up the thinnest women as the most desirable, thus ensuring that psychologically the chains tighten even more.

Of course, there are men with weight problems too, but I don't think they are as crazily obsessed with the problem as women are. Now I'm not suggesting that this is exactly what happened, or even that something must be done about it, I'm just saying IF it is true, it sure would be the most Machiavellian strategy of oppression ever.

Oh My God, Don't Get Me Started On Models

This is one of my favorite stories and it seems kind of appropriate here so I'm sneaking it in. It's not really about dieting, but about manipulating women.

There is a New York writer called Coerte Felske whose books are smart and fascinating and totally pop and horrifying all at once. His first book or the first one that made it big [45] was basically about how to date models. It tells the story of a very shallow guy who in the end lowers his standards and dates a girl who is not a model. Of course, she is heartbreakingly beautiful and *could* be a model, but that's not the point. Anyway, in this book, the main character (who I'm pretty sure is Coerte because the author picture on the back shows a guy who is handsome in that man-about-town way) calls models 'Thing.' As in "Hey look, Thing just walked in the gallery" and other girls 'Civilian' and (I swear I'm getting to the point), during a great conversation, the main character describes to a buddy exactly how you pick up a model.

Here's the technique (masterfully manipulative). You find a bar where models hang out and you wait until a bunch of them come in, then you go over and stand next to the best-looking one, but pretend not to notice her. Hopefully you're near enough to the bar so you can order a drink. Or you can be standing at the jukebox. Anywhere your attention can seem to be occupied by something other than her.

Then, after a minute, you lean kind of casually in her direction, point to another model across the room and say, "That girl is really hot." The model will try not to pout and she will talk to you, but eventually it will get around to, "What about me? Aren't I hot?" Then quite casually, you look her over and proclaim, "You'd be pretty good if you lost five pounds." That model, Coerte assures his buddy, will follow you to the ends of the earth. [46]

[45] The Shallow Man by Coerte Felske

[46] I guess I shouldn't sneer quite so vehemently at models. I mean, it's not their fault and, really, most of them don't CLAIM to be smart so why must I so contemptuously point out that they are not? You know the answer, right? Jealous, okay, I'm jealous.

You can lose five pounds permanently by simply giving up some foods forever.

44

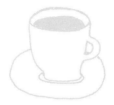

a) Sugar

Cindy was 5'6" and, beginning in high school, usually weighed somewhere between 120 and 150 pounds. Exactly where depended on how she felt: was she in love? did she like her job? where was she living? She got a little fatter when she had her two babies and, truthfully, after the second one, her range was more 135 to 160. (Or 162.) Anyway, her husband loved her and their children, and their children were totally lovely, so she was pretty happy. They lived in Santa Cruz, California near the beach and their lives were nice and relaxed.

Then Cindy read the book <u>Sugar Blues</u> by William Duffy and it scared the pants off her. Also, she hated sugar, so Cindy promptly decided that the whole family should give up sugar and use other sweeteners like rice syrup, bran malt and sometimes maple syrup. That was ten years ago.

Since then, her weight swings have been much lower than they used to be and her energy level is amazing. She's still kind of chunky when she's at the high end but not nearly as bulldozer-like as before and when she's at the low end, she's pretty darned pleased. (See Hint # 37, which also talks about the deadly evil which is sugar.)

b) I gave up cream in my coffee.

This happened when I was about 27 years old, just after I published the book <u>The Guide to The Best Ladies' Bathrooms in Downtown Chicago</u> which I remember because the female journalists all wanted to have coffee with me and then acted like I was hard-bitten for not having cream in my coffee. (Okay, I admit it, having lady journalists think me hard-bitten was pleasurable beyond belief.)

But giving up cream is a bit like giving up salt. At first it seems inconceivable, then, strangely, after you haven't had cream for about two weeks, you will like your black coffee better.

After about a month of coffee with no cream, I lost five pounds without making a single other change. I still swung back and forth between two weights, but instead of 125 to 140, it was now 115 to 135. This doesn't mean I never reached my top weight again but, as it happens, only once or twice since.

More Cream

But while we're on the subject of cream, let me creep even further out on a limb: it's very beneficial to give up dairy completely. Milk is a product that was designed to take a baby cow from 61 pounds to 400 pounds in six months. That's its *purpose*. You should feel completely horrified to put a substance in your mouth that is designed to double your weight in a matter of days. I mean, is milk really that good? I prefer to spend my calories on chocolate. (Okay, I know, it often contains some milk. Maybe I should say: "I prefer to use my dairy on chocolate?")

c) Cheese.

It's basically impossible for me to give up cheese. But I like to *pretend* that I have given up cheese, which means that rather than having cheese for every meal, I only have cheese twice a week. If someone asks me, "Do you want cheese on that?" I say "Oh no," recoiling at the very thought. But then, whenever I get a craving for cheese, I actually go hunting it down in the grocery store, smelling every cheese, figuring out which one I want most. And if I come across one of those cheese sample displays, oh, am I in heaven. But cheese is bad. Yes. Very bad. Hm. I think what I'm saying here is "Don't eat cheese accidentally."

Courtney Love and Cheese

About ten years ago there was an excerpt in *Harper's* from an interview Courtney Love did with Lisa Carver in *Rollerderby #12*, quoting Courtney on the awfulness of cheese and how she'd been a bit of a porker until she gave up cheese, at which point she slimmed right down – didn't have to do anything else. Cheese was a devil food, she said, well, now I'm kind of making this up, but it was all about how she had given up cheese forever and was going to shun cheese for the rest of her life. My friends and I loved the article since we are against cheese ourselves, and were quite interested to see a celebrity also go on record as being a cheese opponent. My friend Helen and I were particularly captivated by the article.

Anyway, time went by, let's say about two years, and my boyfriend and I were invited to a christening party for the child of another rock star, but I decided we couldn't go because Helen and I were in the middle of a fight and it was likely Helen would be at the christening. I thought it was wrong to hastily patch up our differences just to satisfy the expediency of a social situation. So I said to my boyfriend, "I don't care how many celebrities will be there, I love Helen and want the fight to end the right way."

But it turned out I made a big mistake because Helen later told me (our fight was soon settled) that at the party, while everyone was kind of standing around looking cool, Courtney Love came in and pretty much walked right over to Helen and started talking. So they exchanged a few nothing comments and Helen was kind of wishing I was there to tell some stories but then, Courtney Love turned to the hors d'oeuvre table and immediately began eating A LOT OF CHEESE! At that point, Helen really was wishing I'd been there to confront Courtney about her lack of consistency. [47] Outrageous! I mean, here we had been

[47] Sadly, though, it's doubtful I would have said anything. I'm a bit timid and only confrontational if it's an emergency.

thinking that Courtney Love hated cheese as much as we did. (But who knows? Maybe she was just dipping into the verboten food like all mere mortals do from time to time.)

d) Which brings me to bread.

Bread is an extremely delicious food, made even more desirable when I was young because my mother had a rule that we couldn't have bread until we had eaten our entire dinner. She unwittingly made bread equal to dessert. Consequently, my brothers and sisters—and especially me!—are all extremely fond of bread, often clamoring for more and more when we go out to dinner. (In fact, if we are out as a family, the waitress is often stunned to find herself refilling the bread basket a million times and wondering how all this activity will affect her tip.[48]) Bread with non-dairy margarine, or any kind of non-dairy spread, is not that fattening, but it is also, I'm afraid, not that good for you.

Lots of people are allergic to wheat. For years I thought I was not one of them because I thought allergic reactions always result in anaphylactic shock. Hives, red nose, itching, difficulty breathing, plummetting blood pressure and closing off of the

----

48 Tipping. A subject on which, as a former waitress, I have quite a few thoughts. It is very important to tip well. First of all, a tip over 20%, even a very small amount over will be read as high approval. Often this is merely a matter of a dollar or two, sometimes even 50 cents. And what better use can 50 cents ever be put to than increasing someone's self-esteem? Secondly, when someone tips you well, you remember them. Wouldn't you rather have a world full of people who remember you fondly? Again a small price to pay for a large benefit.

Since you've followed me this far into the footnote, I am encouraged to tell you a small waitressing story. My last waitressing job (and my first job in New York) was at The Noho Star. It was quite an eye-opener. Not only were the people significantly more demanding than anyone I'd ever run into before, but I witnessed more disasters in my six months there than I had in my entire previous working history. In no particular order: one of the cooks had an epileptic seizure in the middle of dinner; a customer, while waiting for soup, passed out at the table and cut his head open hitting the floor; a sniper who had taken against the Jewish Defense League caused the entire block to be shut down; but my favorite was when the kitchen caught on fire in the middle of breakfast. I was in the process of asking two rather good-looking guys what kind of toast they wanted when most of the customers ran past me toward the door. Quickly turning towards the kitchen, I saw flames so high they hit the ceiling and fanned out across the rear of the restaurant. I stood there in shock. (You'd think I would have been prepared by then, and you know, maybe I could have handled another sniper or epileptic fit, but this?) One of the cooks grabbed a fire extinguisher and in a matter of minutes put the whole thing out. Almost as soon as it started, it was over. But the strange thing was that during the entire episode about one-third of the customers just went right on eating as if nothing was happening. Also, wonderfully, most of the herd of fleeing customers had tipped me before they fled.

throat. But there is another kind of allergic reaction, which is milder and manifests itself with irritability and then sleep. (It's as if the hives are on the inside.)[49] Alcohol does this to a lot of people, and red wine more so. It makes them argumentative. Bread does the same thing but the reaction to bread is more like a system shutdown. This is very useful to know.[50]

Bread as Valium

Many years ago, in Chicago, I knew a girl named Thea who was small and quite lovely. She was part of the music scene and hung out with musicians and DJs. She had dark hair cut very short and always had on a black leather coat and often red pants with black motorcycle boots. When Thea would feel overwhelmed by the world she would stay home and eat an entire loaf of toasted bread. The only reason I found out about this was that one day, when I ran into her in a club ("950", also known as "Lucky Number"), she started telling me about a very strange coincidence she had just discovered: her boyfriend Lewis's mother, who was manic/depressive, would occasionally eat an entire loaf of toast to calm down. "Just like me," she added.

And calm you down it will. In fact, eat enough bread and you will have a hard time keeping your eyes open. If you are really restless and cannot sleep, eat four whole-wheat bagels, three English muffins, or a pile of rye toast and you will have no problem nodding off. (Actually, the effort of digesting a lot of anything will allow you to sleep, but bread works the best.)

Some Other Foods to Give Up

These four foods—sugar, cream, cheese and bread—are just examples, starting points. There are other foods you can permanently give up that will help. Fried foods. The rest of the dairy family. I, for some reason, find it quite amusing to consider some foods "quite out of the question." I imagine myself a snobby English

[49] Again here I realize I am skating at the far edge of accepted scientific thought.

[50] Learn more about food allergies: Food Allergies and Food Intolerance, by Jonathan Brostoff and Linda Gamlin.

aristocrat from just before the war, secretly looking through her lorgnette at those so crass as to indulge in port, while each evening before the ball, I secretly nip laudanum in my boudoir.

(That, of course, is the lapses.)

45 Read a lot of diet books.

I find them quite inspiring and the inspiration lasts for at least four hours afterwards. So, theoretically, if I read a diet book every four hours I could be very slim. "Slim." Ooooh, I love that word.

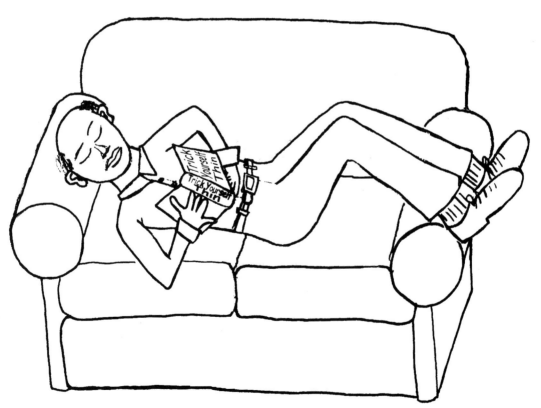

Man sleeps peacefully.

"Svelte." "Lanky."

But of course I don't read that many diet books.[51] Just like chewing each bite fifty times, I forget to do it. But when I remember, I have no problem dieting and, as the fantasy writer Terry Pratchett says, "Of course, it was only a temporary measure, but Rincewind has always considered that life was no more than a series of temporary measures strung together."

Using drugs to lose weight leads to trouble. 46

Yes, it's true that being a drug addict makes you thin. Leaf through any issue of *People* to find one stunning example after another of self-medicating gone badly wrong. But, as my father warned me when I was young, *all* drugs are bad. Even prescription drugs. Try to find an alternative whenever possible. (Okay, I admit the strange tropical disease needed a pile of poisonous antibiotics, but the operative words are "whenever possible." And antibiotics don't exactly get you high.)

Being a drug addict might occasionally look like fun from afar, but it is not. The self-recrimination alone is a thousand times worse than merely being fat. And at least when you are fat you are not actively mean to other people. You probably have rarely stolen to buy food. Or lied . . . Well, forget about that one. Hmmm, rarely stolen. Rarely told someone they were a despicable human or blurted out your real opinion of their competence as a boss because you were high on Oreos. And my guess would be you never had sex with someone deeply embarrassing because you had overeaten. Okay, case closed. No drugs.

Which brings me to a related topic.

51 You might ask: "Jane, you don't read that many diet books compared to whom? Compared to a person who is naturally thin?"

47 All medicine makes you fat.

Even diet medicine. Maybe diet medicine most of all.

Why? Because no matter what medicine you take, eventually you have to stop taking it and when that happens, you swing like a pendulum in the opposite direction. This is simply the way life works: you will always be swinging from side to side. Unfortunately, there is no standing still, no reaching the perfect point and staying there, but the less wild the swings, the less tumultuous the ups and downs, the better off you are. And any thing you ingest besides food causes a wild swing. (And sometimes, as we know, food itself swings you.)

What we're aiming for is a life where the swings are very slight and very slow.

48 Vitamins and other miracles.

Vitamins. I'm pretty sure that antioxidants work. I've tried them on myself and I honestly believe I look better from having taken them. Vitamin C. Vitamin C is essential for the functioning of your body. When you don't get enough, your body will crave more through eating. Lots of Vitamin C. Take at least 3000 mgs a day. Carotene, Vitamin E. But don't just listen to me.

Read up on vitamins [52] and how they should be combined. Take a good multivitamin. The whole-food ones are best. The health food store vitamins are much better than the regular drug store vitamins, which often contain poisonous compounds. Never forget for a second that most manufacturers care absolutely, totally,

52 Prescription for Nutritional Healing: A Practical A-Z Reference to Drug-Free Remedies Using Vitamins, Minerals, Herbs, and Food Supplements by Phyllis A., C.N.C. Balch, James F., M.D. Balch

completely about making money and, no matter what they may say or advertise, not one whit about the welfare of you and me, the little people.

Vitamin Usage Can Also Be Enjoyably Complicated For Those of Us Who Relish That Kind of Thing

Some vitamins need to be taken with other vitamins to be effective. Vitamin C should be taken with bioflavonoids.

A big source of bioflavonoids is orange peels, by the way – in case you want to eat those. I find them quite delicious myself but, as you may remember, my childhood was filled with odd tastes: grass, paper and wool in rather impressive amounts.

> **PAINFUL MEMORY OF MY ODD EATING HABITS.**
> One of my more embarrassing childhood moments was standing in line at the grocery store with my mother and having her yell out, quite annoyed and quite oblivious to the attention she was attracting, "Jane, have you been eating your coat again?!!!" Could I help it that my cashmere coat was quite delicious? So, orange rinds. Yes.

Calcium should be taken in concert with D, magnesium and boron. E is better if there is a variety of tocopherols, not just A-tocopherol. But this information can be quite boring and difficult to keep in one's mind. When I have a problem I want to fix, I look around for someone who is a bit of a health-food-and-vitamin nut. Are they oldish but still looking fabulous? I ask them what I should take and follow their instructions. At the same time, I try to be careful to follow my own instincts and do the mildest form of whatever suggestion is made. For example, since I'm pretty healthy, I don't need six multi-vitamins a day. It's perhaps too early in the evolution of man for us to know exactly what we need. As I always say to my friends, "Don't forget, we're still in the middle of history. We don't know everything yet."

Read and Remember

There is one astounding miracle cure in the vitamin category and that is iron. I don't know if this happens to men, but sometimes women get an attack of iron-poor blood. The first time it happened to me I was working at a publishing house called Thunder's Mouth Press and suddenly I could barely lift a book. I dragged myself around, clutching onto the edges of desks to maneuver about the office, laughing weakly. During my lunch hour I would lie down. It felt like I was sinking into the center of the earth. Day after day this went on, then one day I found myself spontaneously singing the Geritol song (which product, I hear, makes seniors feel peppy not so much from the iron but from its very high alcohol content.)

I thought to myself, "Hey, maybe I need iron." I took an iron pill and felt quite normal—in fact, actually perky—within half an hour.

Another Really Radical Miracle Cure. And, In My Opinion, Funny

Now that I'm on the subject of miracle cures, I must tell you that, regretfully, there aren't that many. Most cures require you to do something day after day, week after week, year after year and then you accrue the most infinitesimal benefit which must be married to some *other* thing that you also must do day after day, etc. until together they make the tiniest difference. (Of course, one of the themes of this book is that a pile of tiny differences can make a very impressive hill, so I'm not saying "there are no miracle cures." I'm just saying they are few and far.)

But but but, all those cautionary notes being sounded, there is a second miracle cure and I can barely contain myself here because the second cure is so disgusting I must beg most of you to stop reading. Now. Skip ahead to the next page and the sub-title 'Narrow Thinking.' Knowing about iron may be miracle cure enough for you.

Okay, if you're still with me, here we go. It's a miracle cure for a sty (an unsightly infection of the eye.) Usually, if you get a sty, it takes a minimum of a week to ten days to rid yourself of it. If you never get sties you probably couldn't care less, but if you do get them, you will be overjoyed to learn there is a cure because they are quite annoying. Okay. Are you ready? Here it is: If you want to cure a sty, when you get up in the morning, put a couple of drops of your own *first urine of the day* in your eye. A couple of drops of urine and it is CURED COMPLETELY in half an hour. (Come to think of it, peeing on a jellyfish sting is also said to effect a pretty miraculous recovery, but that's not exactly an everyday emergency.)

Perhaps you might like to hear the story of how it came to happen that I found this out.

Many years ago, an unsuccessful suitor had given me a health cure book.[53] I read about the urine cure in there, but I had absolutely no intention of ever trying it. But one day, I was sitting with a gaggle of my fellow waitresses in the restaurant where we worked when the universally-feared manager walked by. She had a sty, so I stage-whispered, "Hey, Zöe should try putting a couple drops of urine in her eye." Then I explained about the book, but the only reason I'd said anything was to kind of make fun of her. About three weeks later, one of the other waitresses came up to me and said, "You know that sty cure? It works." "What?" I couldn't imagine what she was talking about. She explained that the crazy cure worked.

Then, about two years later, I myself was afflicted with a sty. I thought 'why not?' and sure enough – miracle cure.

Narrow Thinking Can Ruin Your Life

Always try to keep your mind open: you may acquire new information. While the vast majority of what you hear is complete claptrap, sometimes extremely valuable bits of truth slip through.

....

53 The suitor fell by the wayside after a couple of weeks, but the book stayed with me for years, until finally it, too, was lost.

49 Organic food is better.

Again, remember the principle of "*what you do every day.*" What you do every day does not have an immediate effect, but it does affect how you'll be when you're old, that is – when you *really* need it.

And even if it's not better, organic food gives you a chance to spend more money. Spending money is very good because it makes the person that you are giving the money to happy and then they radiate love toward you. If you recall, tipping is brilliant this way. Remember what I told you: all you have to do is give someone a dollar tip when they usually get fifty cents and they will shower you with love. From an emotional standpoint this is very good and will help you eat better. *And* it is always good to practice being loved; it forces you to learn how to bear it.

Back to the Actual Subject: Organic Food

I actually have absolutely no proof that organic is better except my own appearance. I have eaten organic food whenever possible since I was nineteen. And since that is one of the everyday, day-after-day, facts of my life, I would hate to not mention it when, who knows, it might turn out to be the most important factor in making me look and feel good.

Most essentially, particularly for losing weight: **Organic food tastes better.** Not all the time, just *most* of the time. It is completely beyond me why rich people don't always eat organic food. Especially since you could send your maid to buy it. (Or grow it. Have your maid grow organic vegetables. Now, *that's* rich!)

SOME PSYCHOLOGICAL STUFF

This is totally going overboard and I wouldn't blame you in the slightest if you decided not to read on. Up until this point the book has been about practical tips and hints (okay, with a bunch of crazy digressions, stories and confessions that I warned you about in the first place) on how and when and why and what to eat if you have the three reasons for gaining weight: the need to be the heavy earth-moving machinery, need for padding or the feeling of "not enough." This next part is about how to help untangle the original problems.

Success will make you lose weight. 50

Did you know that if you become successful at least five pounds will simply melt right off? Haven't you ever noticed when a slightly roundish celebrity becomes more famous they lose weight? Kelly Osbourne, Christina Ricci (although she was thin at first as a wee star, then plumped up, then slimmed back down again), Janet Jackson, and, hey, what about Ricki Lake? And this can happen to anyone. In fact (at least I'm hoping), one doesn't really need to become world-famous, you just need to be a little bit more successful in your life to shed those extra spirit-crushing pounds.

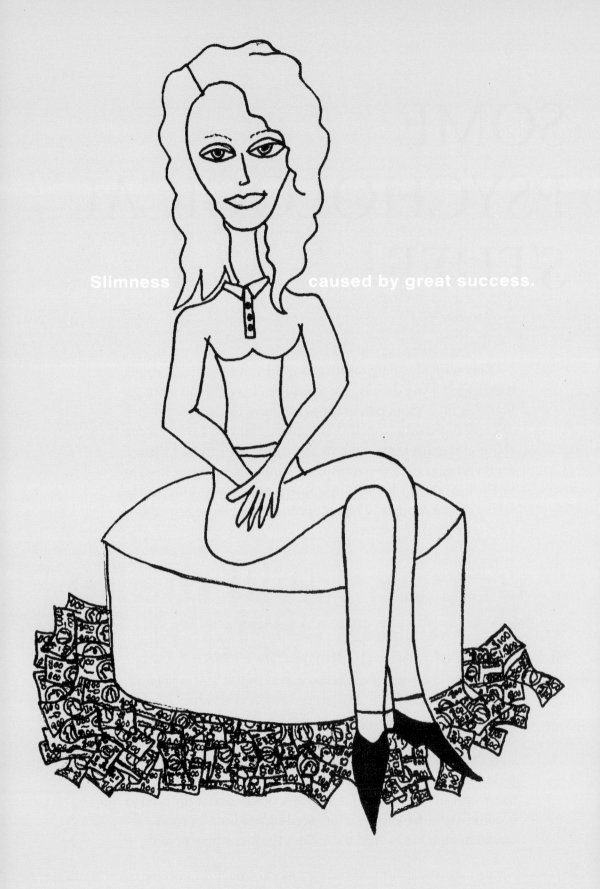

Slimness caused by great success.

The Further Adventures of Rebecca Who Doesn't Eat Sugar

Let's return to the story of the girl who had two jobs in the same building, one working for a stockbroker from 7 am to 11 am, then another upstairs for a lawyer from 11 to 3, then from 3 to 7, back to the stockbroker again. Rebecca.

If you think back to that story, it was while working these jobs that she discovered she was addicted to sugar because if she ate a package of cookies (and I do mean a whole package) or five candy bars (and I do mean five), she would slump back in her chair and murmur "bring it on," no longer caring if she ever got out of the building again. But if she exercised every scrap of self-discipline she possessed and didn't eat the sugar, at 5 p.m., she would be like "GET ME THE HELL OUT OF HERE." Which she considered the far healthier reaction.

But back to the point – which is that when she quit those jobs (at that time, her idea of success), both at once, she went on a car trip to Buffalo, New York with two extremely handsome, brilliant, funny, super-smart guys and the journey was like being in the middle of the most spectacular stand-up comedy routine of all time. She laughed for five days straight. Her stomach hurt, her jaw hurt and ten pounds DISAPPEARED without her having to make any effort whatsoever.

Which she said was lucky since working for two bosses had packed on more, much more, than enough, padding.

Lesson here? Laughing is success.

Side Effects of Getting Thinner To Prepare For

SMALL MEALS MEAN LIGHT SLEEP.

I mentioned this briefly in hint #11, about sleeping. So keep it in mind. When I want to sleep very lightly, I don't eat much the day before. Which is a bit like something I read when I was about eight years old: that Native Americans used the urge to pee as an alarm clock. They knew exactly how much to drink before they went to bed to wake themselves up at specific times. When I read this I got deeply anxious that if I drank too much, I would have to get up in the middle of the night. So I became obsessed before going to bed, as if I were going on a bus trip without an on-board toilet.

My friend Catherine [54] was a painter who had just moved to England, where she was not able to work legally. After a bit of searching, she got hired as a security guard, a job about which she was very excited for two reasons. One was that she was down to about £10 when she was hired, and second, the job was perfect. It paid cash and all she had to do was, twice each hour, walk around the abandoned car dealership she was guarding, mainly to prevent vandalism. At all other times, she was free to read, draw, watch TV, exercise – in fact, do whatever she wanted to do as long as she stayed on the property.

The only problem was that she had to get up at 4 a.m. to get to work on time and didn't have £10 for an alarm clock, she needed it for the bus fare. So she went on a very strict (and economical) diet of fruits and vegetables and found that if she stopped eating at around six at night, she easily popped awake, quite a bit before dawn. One night she made the mistake of eating a large meal at midnight and had a much more difficult time dragging herself from her warm and comfortable bed.

Another Side Effect of Eating Lightly: People Will Pay a Lot More Attention to You.

They will look at you a lot more. This seem desirable, but it's not always so. When you look good, you are much more prominently on view. When you steal a second goody bag, for example, it will be noticed. When you make a snide remark, people will hear it and know that you meant it to be snide. Men will harass you. You have to know in advance that this will happen. Be prepared *before you lose the weight*, otherwise it will scare you. Don't worry about the men. One of the great pleasures of being thin is that when men harass you, you can be cynically witty and they will simply laugh in a jolly way, as if you were kidding. (I like men, but let's face it, the nickname I use—"Mr. Man," is short for "Mr. Young Fellow Who Does Not Notice

54 Yes, you guessed it.
Me again.

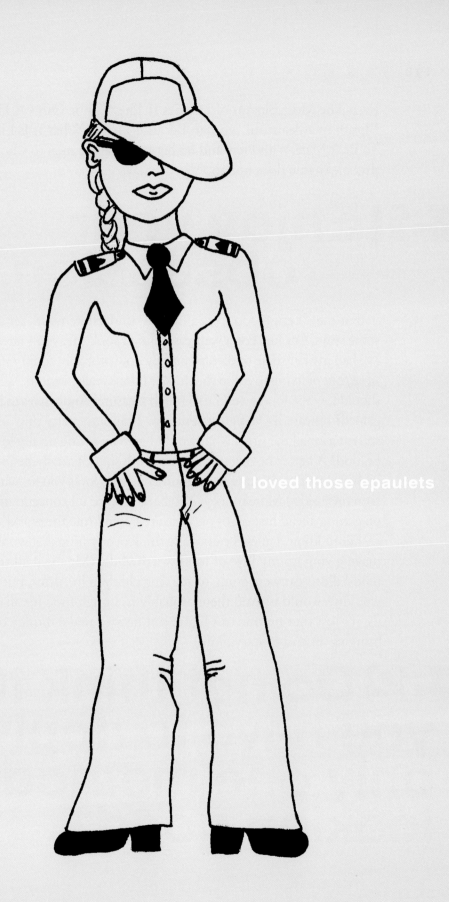

I loved those epaulets

Even The Most Blatant of Idiocies If They Come Out Of The Mouth of a Beautiful Woman Because That Is What It Is Like To Be A Man"—and few and far between are the men to whom that nickname does not apply.

51 Enjoy your obsession.

For me, "I enjoy food," is a massive understatement. Yet, in some ways, I'm kind of a well-disciplined soul. Heaven knows, I've had my fair share of therapy and by now probably could *train myself* out of liking to eat so much. But I don't really want to. Why should I, when food gives me so much pleasure? And what's to be gained? I mean, if I've figured out how I can stay pretty thin and still eat a lot all the time, what would I gain by giving up my love of food? A better boyfriend? I don't think so. (I actually believe in the romantic notion of having someone who loves you for what is on the inside.) More money? Maybe so. Maybe if I concentrated on getting ahead instead of on pleasure I could rule the world.

I don't know. I guess I can't really think of anything that would make giving up my love of food worthwhile. (Maybe if all the food I didn't eat were going to starving children in Africa, but it wouldn't, would it? And there probably *is* enough food for all of us, it's just that no one can figure out how to make money on bringing an end to starvation.)

52 Do not think that you have to apply only one method of looking good.

Apply as many as you like. I believe in applying as many of these hints as I can.

When I was about forty, just before I started getting collagen injections to get rid of the lines on the sides of my mouth, I was telling my friend Kit that I was thinking of doing it. She said, "We have a woman in our yoga class who's in her early fifties and she doesn't have a line on her face. Why don't you just do your yoga?" and I immediately said (and it was unlike me to think of an answer so quickly, usually the most brilliant rejoinder occurs to me four hours later when I'm in the bath) "I want yoga *and* plastic surgery. I want ALL the solutions. I want yoga and a good diet and plastic surgery and therapy and meditating and my horoscope read and massage and walking and psychic consultation. You got it? I want it."[55]

This same principle can be applied to dieting. Don't just try one technique, pile them all on top of one another. Do one for four hours, then try something else. All strung together, you'll have made a pearl necklace, a knit sweater, a brick wall.

Therapy is totally fun. 53

Think about it. Once a week you get to go and tell someone everything you truly think. With no repercussions. It is *completely* about you, the other person never (or rarely) butts in to say what happened to them or even to give their opinion or advice and on top of that, the person is totally on your side. It's funny that some people are so against it. It's beyond funny, in fact. It's incomprehensible. Here's how I think of it: it's as if apple pie[56] were suddenly invented and a small amount of people in the world tried it and they all said: "WOW, this apple pie stuff is really good." But

[55] I'm a glutton.
(In case you hadn't noticed.)

[56] Okay. That's probably a bad example to use in a diet book, so let's say it's apple pie sweetened with maple syrup and you've been really good on your diet for a long time and really don't need to lose any more weight.)

almost everyone else-—most of the rest of the world, in fact—
said, "WE WILL NEVER TRY APPLE PIE BECAUSE WE
KNOW IT IS TERRIBLE." And then, a very good and trusted
friend, who has tried the apple pie, says, "No really, you should
try it. I tried it and I thought it was one of the most delicious tastes
ever." But the world stands its ground and shouts: "I WOULD
RATHER DIE BEFORE I TRIED APPLE PIE!"

You get my point. Even a bad therapist is fun, and a great one
is totally magical.

Remember, beauty is a direct by-product of health. Not just
physical health but mental health, too. That's why we revere
beauty so much. Far from being a sign of shallowness (as I
thought, snippily, well into my twenties) our love of beauty is
a regard for the glory of what being human, at its best, is.

Only one caveat. Do *not* have sex with your therapist. Ever. It
is much worse than having sex with your mother. In fact, if you
find yourself in a situation in which you might be about to have
sex with your therapist or, more to the point, that your therapist is
about to have sex with you, have sex with your mother first so you
can experience some small portion of how badly it is going to make
you feel.

54 How you look at life is what it is.

This is true in two different ways.

I have a friend named Mark who lives in Los Angeles and sees
the world in very dark terms. If you're thinking about going to
29 Palms, he'll tell you there's bound to be a lot of traffic and the
trip there will be tedious. If you think you might get a good job
as a magazine writer, he'll be sure to inform you that that kind of
job is insecure, that your writing may be faddish for a while,
but then your style will fall out of favor and you'll be back on the
street again.

Mark is funny and charming and when he was young he was unbelievably beautiful but now he lives in a charmless, crumbling duplex and works as a secretary for a temp service. He is divorced from a wife with whom he was never in love, has two kids he doesn't think much of, and spends his free time going to flea markets because he thinks it's a waste to furnish his house (or life) expensively. At one point, Mark very much wanted to date me and I considered it because he was quite kind and like I said, funny, but in the end, there was no way. I couldn't be sure if my view of life would be stronger than his and I am convinced that, if I were to accidentally catch his pessimism, my life would be ruined.

Because if you see your life as glorious and each second of every day as an amazing and interesting event that might, in turn, lead to other amazing and interesting events, then two things happen. First of all, you *are* having a good life, because that is how you are experiencing it. But on top of that, if you approach life this way, then all kinds of amazing and interesting events actually *do* happen.

Never give up your dreams. 55

There are no self-help books, no religious texts, no romance fix-its, no great novels that do not say this exact thing. The Alchemist, The Celestine Prophecy, Holes, *Star Wars, Erin Brokovich, The Matrix,* in fact, just about every Hollywood movie ever made.

That doesn't mean you can't ever change to another dream. That's okay. All rock stars wanted to be baseball players when they were young but they injured themselves and had to settle for international musical fame with hot and cold running women instead. Sometimes fate changes your dream for you, like maybe when you were young you wanted to be a dancer, but when you got to

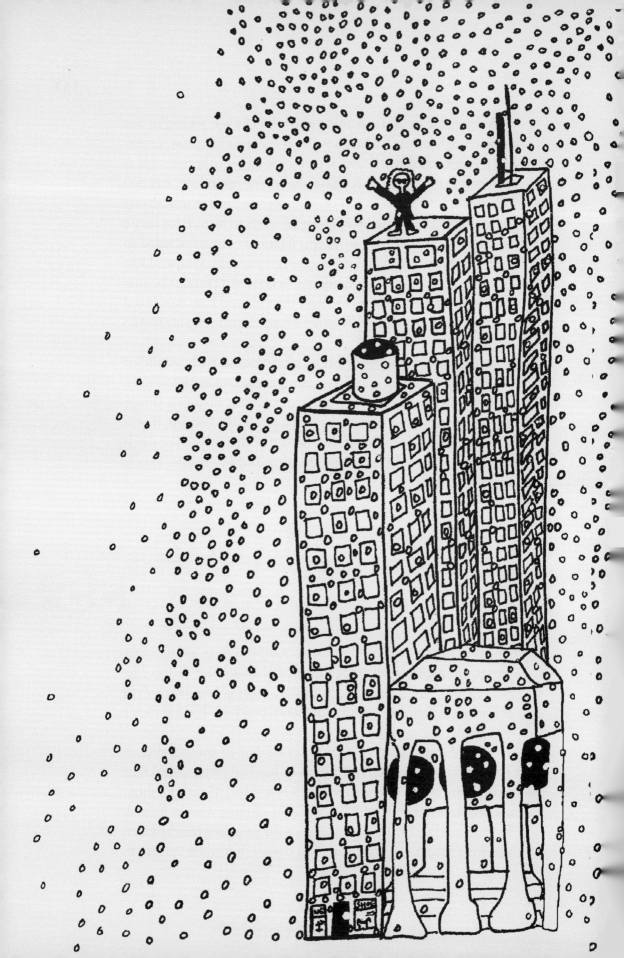

be about thirteen you grew just a bit too tall to be chosen for the premier roles. Or your breasts got too big. Or you got interested in boys. Or your schoolwork got harder. So you started thinking about giving up your dream.

Don't do it. *Do not give up.* Fate may prevent your dream from coming true. So what? Change your dream. Dream of being a choreographer instead. Even if it takes fifty years, it'll be worth it. Or the hell with it, keep trying to be a dancer. Who cares whether you get there or not? If you pursue your dream throughout an entire lifetime, the mere fact of your pursuit will protect you from mediocrity. I promise.

**This is the most important hint in the book
and that is why it is quietly hidden here in the end.
It might be possible that by following this one maxim,
my life has changed completely.
Here it is:**

If I am afraid of something, the rule is: I must do It. 56

This means that if the thought of performing an action frightens me and I see other people doing it—sometimes easily—I MUST DO THAT ACTION.[57]

When I was in grammar school, my father, a surgeon, was training me to be a doctor. He would take me to operations in the middle of the night and tell me stories of medical triumphs and disasters. Unfortunately I was the sort of child who was obsessed with disaster. One day he told me the story of a

[57] This does not include totally unreasonable acts like running naked through a dangerous neighborhood at 3 a.m., or illegal acts, like robbing a bank or running every red light on your way to work.

girl who had come over from Bulgaria with her father. Her mother had died when she was quite young and the two of them had made their way to the new world together. The father slaved on an assembly line and devoted his entire life to his daughter. And what a spectacular daughter she turned out to be. Incredibly gorgeous and smart as greased lightning. She went to Harvard and graduated with every honor. Her father was proud beyond description. But the summer after she graduated, she and her trust fund boyfriend went on a motorcycle trip across the country. Late one night they got into a terrible accident with a drunk driver. The girl suffered extensive head trauma that left her a vegetable for the rest of her life.

This story completely freaked me out. I never wanted to be in control of a car. Ever.

For years, people had to drive me around. Many many people tried to teach me how to drive. A couple of times people actually gave me cars, hoping that would force me into learning.

But eventually I came to realize that because I was deathly afraid of driving, it was completely imperative that I learn to drive.

Just before I moved to New Mexico, my cousin Tom suggested that I take driving lessons in Chicago because he thought it was better to learn to drive in a city. For some reason I listened to him. My teacher was an elderly Philipino man. He was quite supportive of my driving, although once he did say I drove awfully fast for a person who didn't know how to drive. I told him that I didn't *want* to drive fast, but my whole family drives fast and something in my body seems to insist that I do so too.

For a long time I continued to be frightened when I drove, but that didn't matter to me. What mattered was that *I was driving*. I could *drive*. I could get in a car and go to a new place. Later, when I got a credit card, I could *rent* a car, so even though I didn't own a car, I could still get behind the wheel of one and drive anywhere I wanted. Once I rented a car in Guatemala and drove to Costa Rica. How completely totally, amazingly marvelous was that? It was as if I had become an entirely different person. A better person, stronger and more courageous.

Another thing I was always afraid of was any contact with large sums of money. For years I waitressed – usually at the best place in town, and basically lived on cash. I had enough for my simple needs, but it was not clear that I would ever be able to buy anything expensive. I don't think I ever even bought a tv. When I was 38, I got married. I got married for two reasons:

1. I had a boyfriend who insisted.
2. I was at a point in therapy where my therapist was suggesting that my lack of desire to marry might stem from a fear of commitment, rather than from what I had always thought of as a feminist political stance.

Anyway, my husband—quite generous, frightfully intelligent and a big risk-taker—was just starting a business. About half a year into the marriage, in one month, he ran up charge card debt of $22,000. When I opened the envelope and saw the amount, I felt like I'd been dropped from a ten-story building. What the heavens-to-murgatroyd was I going to do? And we're not talking Visa, we're talking American Express (outstanding balance payable in full).

As it turned out, I managed to raise that sum and pay the bill. Aside from the fright, everything was fine. My feeling now is that one of the greatest things I took from that marriage was confidence in my ability to deal with large sums of money.

More More More, More About Me. Oh, How I Wish You Were Here To Tell Me Stories About You (But I'm Almost Through)

Now this might be hard to believe from what you've read thus far, but I am actually a deeply timid person. Why I am not an old maid with mousy brown hair pulled back in a bun, working as a librarian in some small safe town, spending evenings at home watching soap operas taped on my old cranky VCR is beyond me.

Once a temp agency got me work for some reinsurance brokers on Wall Street. I was one of three girls doing contract assembling and typing for an entire department and we were killing ourselves every day. The two other girls were whip-smart and the brokers were taking advantage of the superior type of help they had.

When I asked Rhoda at the employment agency if I could leave because the brokers were so abusive, she said "Can you hold on until I find a replacement?" I agreed. But week after week no replacement was found. Finally I figured it out. The brokers were extremely reluctant to hire a replacement for me. Why should they? I was working my tush off for very little pay.

At the same time as I was being totally oppressed, I was advising my friends (who at that stage in their careers were moving from middle management to vice presidencies or editorships) to go in and tell their bosses they needed a raise or promotion.

I finally decided it was time to practice what I was preaching. I called Rhoda to tell her I was going to ask for a raise. I determined to go to the head broker, a formidable giant of a man named John, and tell him that if he wanted to keep me working there, he'd have to pay me $300 a week on top of the money that was going to the temp agency. I was completely terrified the entire day, trembling really, faint with fear and I almost chickened out, but at three, when he came back from lunch, I walked into his office.

The guy was completely flabbergasted. "I'm going to call your agency and tell them you're doing this," he threatened.

"They already know," I said.

"Well," he stalled, at a loss for words. "I have to ask the head of human resources."

"Okay," I said, about a thousand times more calmly than I felt inside. "Just let me know by the end of the day."

At the end of the day, he called me into his office. "The head of human resources said we were not able to meet your salary requirements and so you can go at the end of the week."

"Oh no," I said. "If you cannot meet my salary requirements, I am leaving at the end of the day."

You cannot begin to imagine how profound an effect this encounter had on me. I mean it was win/win for me since I didn't want to be there anyway, but heck, the feeling I had after I actually went in and confronted him was so **empowering**. Suddenly I saw myself as a daredevil, afraid of nothing. And best of all, my courage had gotten me out of a terrible situation. When, at the end of the day, I walked

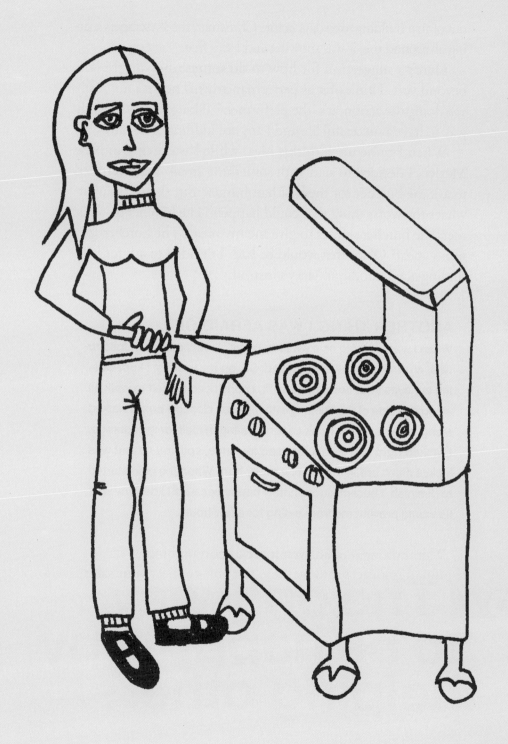

If you like to cook, cook large meals for other people.

out of that building, two days before Christmas, the skyscrapers soaring all around me, it was snowing and I was free.

Here's a suggestion for how to do something you think is beyond you. Think of it as performance art. Then it's not really *you* doing the action, it's "the performer." Taking risks is the only way to have a successful life and I am not kidding. The only way.

When I came up with this idea, while I was living in New Mexico, I decided to start with something small. Was I terrified to ask the butcher for the best hamburger? But then I thought: what's the worst thing that could happen? The butcher glares at me? The butcher refuses to give me my meat? The butcher *spits* in my meat? Okay, that would be bad. I decided to ask for help finding a red hoodie at Macy's instead.

ANOTHER THING I WAS AFRAID OF

When I was working as a security guard, I realized I was afraid to walk around with my eyes closed. So, on my rounds, I kept closing my eyes and, during one shift, I convinced myself to walk all along one side of the building with my eyes closed. I boldly walked along, and just when I was congratulating myself for my courage, I walked right into a pole, bruised my knee, split my lip and was lucky I didn't break my nose. It really hurt. When the pain started to diminish, I became inordinately happy because I knew my split lip would prevent me from eating for a few hours.

Wait. I thought of an even more important hint:

57 The only way to be happy is by helping others.

I might have to write a whole book on this one.

And last, but least of all least:

Compliment yourself constantly, night and day.   58

Your brain has an entire section that does nothing but talk to itself all the time. Which would be merely an interesting curiosity, except that *you believe what it says.* And the things you are saying to yourself are quite often discouraging things like "I'm so fat" or "Why am I so stupid?" or "I hate him, I hate him, I hate him."

So if your brain is playing a negative tape, it's time to replace the bad tape with a better one, saying something a little more encouraging, like my current favorite, "I am a spectacular being."

At first, it's difficult because of course it's easier to play the same old tapes. (Just like in real life, playing the same tape over and over is easier than searching for and inserting a new one.) Also, I didn't want to recite corny slogans all day. I found that saying things to myself like "You, Jane, are a spectacular being" quite embarrassing, even to myself. But then I got over it. And when I got used to doing it, I found the transformation that occurred was enormous. Now I can quite happily chant things like "I am very very rich" or "I love you, Jane" while walking down the street, riding a bus or driving in my car. You get used to change if you keep working at it.

For example: when my mother was about eight she was sent to a camp in Maine that had at one time enjoyed a rather sterling reputation. Unbeknownst to my mother's family, whose information was a bit out-of-date, the camp had become popular with the sons and daughters of New York City psychiatrists. My mother's first week at the camp was quite terrifying. Almost all the other kids had neuroses of gargantuan proportions, some screaming all night long, others throwing their food, many engaged in rampant kleptomania and self-mutilation. Also, every morning at 6 a.m., everyone in the camp, counselors included, was required to run, nude, down to the freezing cold lake and jump in. But my mother said that after a week or so, this all became quite normal to her and she was no longer bothered in the slightest. It was only when she got back to St. Louis and was re-introduced to "normal life" that she saw how far outside the usual boundaries of acceptable behavior she had spent the summer.

The moral of the story is this: Since you can get used to anything, you can even get used to saying nice things to yourself.

How to Make Your Life Wonderful

I've hung out with all levels of society – from movie stars to . . . (now who would I pick at the other end of the social spectrum? Heroin addicts in Chicago? Hispanic waitresses in Albuquerque, New Mexico? Security guards in Oxford, England? Soldiers in Spain? I actually found all these groups every bit the equal, and in many cases the superiors, of the movie stars.) Everyone has the potential for intelligence, beauty and greatness, but some people have a better opinion of themselves which gives them the courage to improve. That's the intrinsic difference. Think of yourself as great. And then act that way.

Me At My Best

I try to see my life as a whole and to concentrate on the times when I was thin. No matter how roundish I may be at any given moment, I force myself to remember: there *were* thin times. **That, too, was me.** And there's no reason that can't be me again. I just have to be ready to handle the flightiness, vulnerability and excitement that comes whenever I'm more pared down.

CONCLUSION

That's about it. It's only a few ideas but I found that by incorporating these hints into my daily life, I gradually became thinner, stayed thinner and best of all, still get to enjoy food A LOT.

Let's go over the hints once again, or rules if you prefer to call them that. (Some people love rules. I have to say that although I'm against authority, I am one of the rule lovers. Particularly rules I have imposed myself.)

So, for example, I often say (as you now know), "I'm against cheese." Once I went to a mall in the small town where I grew up with my nephews. After we had shopped for a while (oh yeah, I remember, it was Christmas), I asked if they wanted anything to eat. "Pizza," they said. So I bought them pizza. "Aren't you going to have any, Jane?" they asked. "No," I said. "I'm against cheese." They both didn't say anything and that seemed to be the end of the matter. But when my brother, their dad, came to pick us up, we got in the van and right away they started jumping up and down excitedly, "Dad, Dad," they said. "Did you know that Jane is against cheese?" My brother thought about that for one second and then in his very calm, dry way said, "Well, let's hope Jane wins."

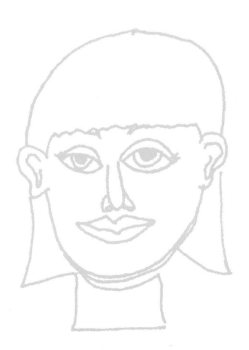
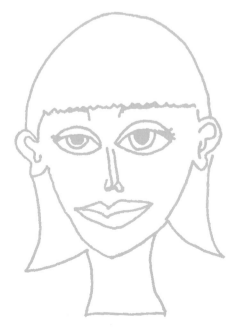

But enough jokes, the hints:

Hints

1. Start Again Every Day.
2. Food Combining Totally Works.
3. Try Not To Eat Before Going To Bed.
4. Eating Vegetables Is A Great Idea.
5. Don't Eat When You Don't Feel Like It.
6. Exercise Is King.
7. Anorexia Is A Bad Idea.
8. Never Try To Discipline Yourself For More Than Four Hours At A Time.
9. Don't Get Bored.
10. Drink Lots Of Water.
11. Sleep.
12. Always Eat Exactly What You Want.
13. Always Eat Food That Tastes Good.
14. It's Totally Worth It To Go To A Lot Of Trouble To Get Exactly What You Want To Eat.
15. Try to Eat in Relaxing Circumstances.
16. Food Made By Someone Who Loves You Is The Food That Is Best.
17. Figure Out What Other Activities Are Pleasures.
18. Then Make A List Of Things That Make Eating A Distant Memory.
19. Next, Figure Out Which Activities Are Most Associated With Eating.
20. Postpone Eating.
21. Set Deadlines.
22. Take Some Foods That Are Normally Thought Of As Diet Foods And Imagine That They Are Forbidden.
23. Sometimes Eating Just Has To Do With The Fun Of Chewing And Swallowing.
24. Don't Drink Anything With Calories.
25. Don't Lie About How Much You've Eaten.
26. Shop For Clothes.
27. Don't Sit Down To Eat At A Party Thinking To Be On A Diet.
28. Try Not To Obsess About Food.
29. Juice Is A Great Invention.

30. It Is Best To Eat Fruit, By Itself, First Thing In The Morning.
31. Make an Attempt To Chew Each Bite Fifty Times.
32. Having A Slow Metabolism Is Not Completely Bad.
33. There Is A Size That Your Body Wants To Be.
34. For Two Weeks Out Of Every Month My Body Likes To Be Fatter And Will Insist I Eat More.
35. When You Get A Craving, Particularly For A Food Considered Healthy, Pay Attention.
36. Never Never Ever Ever Weigh Yourself.
37. Bouillon.
38. When Driving Across The Country, Go To The Grocery Store.
39. Always Have Some Food With You.
40. Candy Is Fattening And Bad For Everyone, Including Small Children and Very Thin People.
41. Yogurt Is Fattening.
42. Keep Away From Salt.
43. Fat On The Other Hand Is Not All Bad.
44. Using Drugs As A Diet Aid Leads to Trouble.
45. All Medicine Makes You Fat.
46. Read A Lot Of Diet Books.
47. Permanently Lose Weight Simply By Giving Up Some Food Forever.

Advanced Secrets

48. Vitamins And Other Miracles.
49. Organic Food Is Better.
50. Success Will Make You Lose Weight.
51. Enjoy Your Obsession.
52. Do Not Think That You Have To Apply Only One Method Of Looking Good.
53. How You Look At Life Is What It Is.
54. Therapy Is Totally Fun.
55. Never Give Up Your Dreams.
56. If I Am Afraid Of Something, The Rule Is: " I Must Do It."
57. The Only Way To Be Happy is By Helping Other People.
58. Compliment Yourself Constantly, Night And Day.

A Don't

Don't go to a country with food that tastes bad. You will wind up eating more and more trying to be satisfied. This is to be distinguished from a country with 'dangerous' food – that is, food that will make you sick. That's okay. The danger will inspire you to eat sparingly and that will help lessen the possibility of acquiring a strange tropical disease of your own. Dangerous stuff (parasites are the first things that comes to mind here) are eliminated more easily if your digestive system is not overburdened.

Bad Diet
Alert

A Couple of Bad Diets

These are examples of eating styles I don't recommend.

THE LA GIRL DIET: STAY COLD!

This is a story from when I first moved to Los Angeles[58] and how I learned what young girls there do to lose weight. They are all impossibly thin and no one in that city ever gets any exercise of any kind, unless you count kissing ass and ruthlessly pushing friends aside and occasionally killing a couple of family members to get to the head of the pack as exercise.[59]

It was New Year's Eve. I was at a party up in the

[58] My job, novel writer, was a beautiful one to have in that city because once I revealed what I did, everyone immediately relaxed: I wasn't dangerous, I wasn't a rival, I wasn't powerful or useful or connected.

[59] Yes, some people in L.A. go to health clubs, but not the hip.

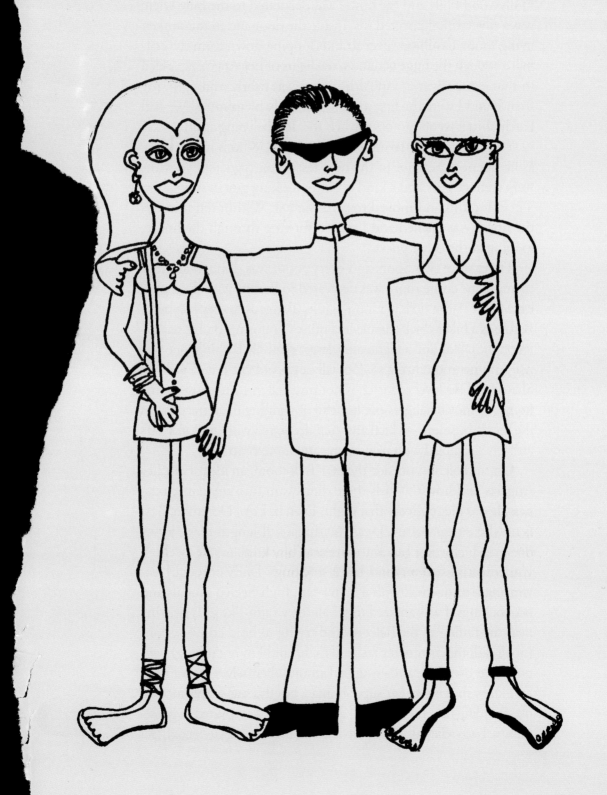

Hollywood Hills and the house was decorated to the hilt. There was a silver, tinsel-covered tree inside the door and in the sunken living room, a million silver strands looping down from the ceiling. Through the huge windows, the lights of Los Angeles sparkled in that same silver color. Although it was nearly midnight, my friends and I were the first to arrive but only by minutes. We had barely shrugged off our coats when the doorbell rang again.

The very fey host twinkled to the door. "Who is it?" he sang, as he opened the door to the next festive partygoers, two stunning teenage girls and a kind of slimy-looking guy in sunglasses. They slunk in and moved toward the bar. Within ten minutes the house was packed and I started moving through the house, looking at the other guests.

There were two floors and every room was done in another theme. One entire room was dedicated to Barbie, with three glass cases full of Barbie dolls in various outfits (Barbie as Audrey Hepburn, Barbie as a biker chick, Barbie in a nurse's uniform), Barbie scenarios on the tables, and a frightening, larger-than-life Barbie in one corner. Another room had a six-foot tall cardboard cut-out of William Shatner. (This level of kitsch is not unusual in L.A. houses—the homes of movie hangers-on, hopeful of winning the lottery that is the movie business—which are often decorated with '50's and '60's artifacts assembled with painstaking attention to detail.)

On the balcony, outside the Star Trek room, an idea about Los Angeles and how the girls there diet swam into my consciousness. It was plenty frosty that night. Even in L.A., December 31st is nowhere near balmy. I was wearing a full-length black jersey dress and over it a black t-shirt and black cashmere sweater. Underneath I had on thick black stockings. Every other girl was wearing a mini-dress with a halter top, high-heeled sandals and no stockings. I was amazed to see all the wraith-like girls swaying near the railing of the balcony and trying to hold conversations (not a skill that is much practiced there, and I'm not joking) with only their own bare arms wrapped around themselves for warmth.

I knew the girls *looked* super-human, but this was simply incredible. Standing near me, I noticed a blonde who was covered in goosebumps. I was relieved. They weren't aliens, they actually *were* cold. But then what could be the reason for dressing so inadequately? Did they think that was the only way to attract men? Possibly. Or maybe they were too stupid to realize that if it was cold, you put on more clothes. But no, I had talked to some of them and they were not *that* dumb. (Not that amusing maybe, but not stupid.) What could it be?

Then it came to me in a flash. They were *dieting*. They lived in an environment where they were required to weigh almost nothing or they would not be considered viable and yet, they never got any exercise. Ever. If you are desperately cold every night, your body will burn calories for heat. That and starving themselves is the L.A. girl diet. Crazy.

Of course, this is not an approach you would want to put into practice in your own life. Just because it might *work* is not enough to say, justify dashing around downtown Chicago in February wearing a t-shirt. But the theory does give me a reason to be happy when I am slightly cold. 'Well, I guess I'm losing weight,' I now think to myself as I shiver my calories away.

Losing Weight By Being Too Hot

And curiously enough, the *opposite* is also true. In my high school there was a brief fad for mail-order plastic suits. When they arrived, you'd put them on and blow them up around you, looking kind of like a transparent Michelin Man. The theory was that sweating would cause you to lose water weight. So, early in life, I encountered the idea that being *hot* makes you lose weight, and I embraced the concept with open and eager plastic-covered arms. And I do believe that a tiny bit of sweat today is a small price to pay for trimmer thighs tomorrow. So whenever I'm hot, I cheerily think, 'Well, how great. I'm losing weight.'

Which, as I just said, I also do when cold. Hot or cold. Either one. Both great.

I Was Tempted To Tell You Another Really Bad Diet Story But Decided Not To

When I was growing up, my mother was a full-on fashion plate. She was (unlike me) tall, slender and clothes draped beautifully on her 5'8" frame. She had thick straight dark hair and was completely natural. Elegant is a word invented for her. Both my parents were chic without trying, their every move graceful and seemingly effortless.

My mother could eat whatever she liked and still stay thin. She was a great cook and threw glamorous dinner parties with artists, doctors and professors. Her sense of color was exquisite and she would be dressed in a Pucci shift with strappy sandals, wielding a spatula and telling a witty story, with the elaborate abundance of the California vegetation as her backdrop. We lived in the country and during the day, my mother often wore tennis shorts with a baggy sweater and tennis shoes. She looked good.

Then one day, things changed. My mother got round, then a bit rounder. She discovered diets, but never really went on one – she loved cheese, pasta, chocolate and her favorite food was bacon.

Just last year, she started to lose weight. Terribly worried, we rushed from all corners of the globe to see what was the matter.

When I arrived at the airport, I walked down the grey corridor when suddenly, there was my mother. At the first sight of her, my breath was taken away. She has white hair that shines like diamonds, she was wearing asparagus green pants which dragged slightly on the ground in a nod to hip-hop, a very pale pink trenchcoat and a deep maroon vintage Calvin Klein sweater.

"Mom," I said.

"Jane!" she beamed. She knew what I was saying and basked.

"What happened? You look great."

"I know." She paused. "Thank you for saying so. That's one of the problems of getting old. No one ever tells you how good you look when you get thin."

She was fine. Just thin again. Just so beautiful. Secretly I chalk up the new thinness to the fact that she had an early read of this book, but who knows? She claims she just finally learned the secret of small helpings. And sure enough, I spent a week with her and the portions she consumed were astoundingly commendable.

Whatever the reason, the story shows that there's hope. That no matter how long you've been a roundish person or how round you've gotten, you can be thin again. Remember, these are the watchwords: experiment and *anything is possible.*

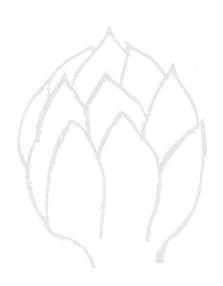

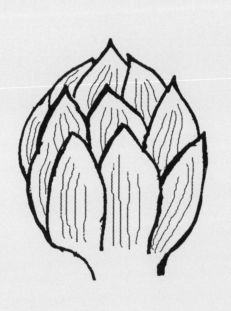

ANOTHER CONCLUSION

Okay. I have many more ideas, but that's enough for now.

It's definitely impossible for me to practice every hint every day. To take all the vitamins, do all the exercises, do all the crazy evasive steps I've devised to keep myself thin would take about forty hours a day, so instead I pick which I feel like that day. Some days I do none. Though by now, I have to say, I'm usually working at least a couple of hints every day. The more I work at it, the more I actually enjoy doing the work. As time goes on, more and more I try to cultivate a *love* of work. The alternative is to just let the whole mess slide into disintegration and decay. Which I know must happen anyway at some point, but when? When is the right time? 60? 70? 80? 90? The later, the better, I say.

It's a lot of slogging away, but when I feel overwhelmed, I say, "If I've done it once, I can do again." Once I lost the first five pounds, I knew the process and I know how to repeat it. By this point in my life I don't panic when I gain weight. I mean, of course, I panic a little bit, that's a motivator, but I'm pretty sure I can take that weight back off. Doing something I've already done is not that hard. It's the new stuff that scares the pants off me.

As I practiced these hints more and more, my tastes changed. Now I no longer like potato chips (repulsively greasy), or candy (too sweet; so sweet it tastes chemical). So try it out, practice the hints and you'll see. One day you'll simply laugh at how beautiful, strong, and happily good you feel. How free and loved. How confident. How capable. How right. How alive. How wonderful. (Not every second, of course, but for a really huge chunk of the time.) And that is a marvelous thing because then the promise of this book will come true: you can eat all you want and still stay thin. And that, my friends, will be enough.

Jane

Further Resources

Books that are not so funny but do expand upon the scientific basis behind some of my ideas.

ALLERGIES
Food Allergies and Food Intolerance, by Jonathan Brostoff & Linda Gamlin

BODY TYPING
Eat Right for Your Type, by Peter J. D'Adamo & Catherine Whitney

CHEWING
The Mayo Clinic on Digestive Health

ENEMAS
A Cancer Therapy: Results of Fifty Cases and the Cure of Advanced Cancer, by Dr. Max Gerso

FOOD COMBINING
Food Combining Bible, by Jan Dries
The Complete Book of Food Combining, by Jan & Inge Dries
Food Combining Made Easy, by Herbert M. Shelton
The Hay Diet Made Easy, by Jackie & Alexandra Habgood

FRENCH FRIES AND OTHER BAD FOODS
Fast Food Nation, by Eric Schlosser

GENERAL WEIGHT LOSS
Fit For Life, by Harvey & Marilyn Diamond

JUICE
Juicing For Life, by Cherie Calbom & Maureen Keane

METABOLISM
The Nutrition Solution: A Guide To Your Metabolic Type, by Harold Kristal

SKIN
The Perricone Prescription, by Nicholas Perricone

SUGAR
Sugar Blues, by William Duffy
Lick the Sugar Habit, By Nancy Appleton, PhD

UNDERSTANDING CRAVINGS
The Diet Cure, by Julia Ross

VEGETABLES
Vegetarian Cooking for Everyone, by Deborah Madison

YOUR LIVER
The Fat Flush Plan, by Ann Louise Gittelman

VITAMINS
Prescription for Nutritional Healing A-To-Z Guide to Supplements: A Handy Resource to Today's
ost Effective Nutritional Supplements
mes F., Md. Balch, Phyllis A. Balch

w that there's usually a lot more information (like publishing dates), but why?
005, this is more than enough information for you to get your hands on these
s.

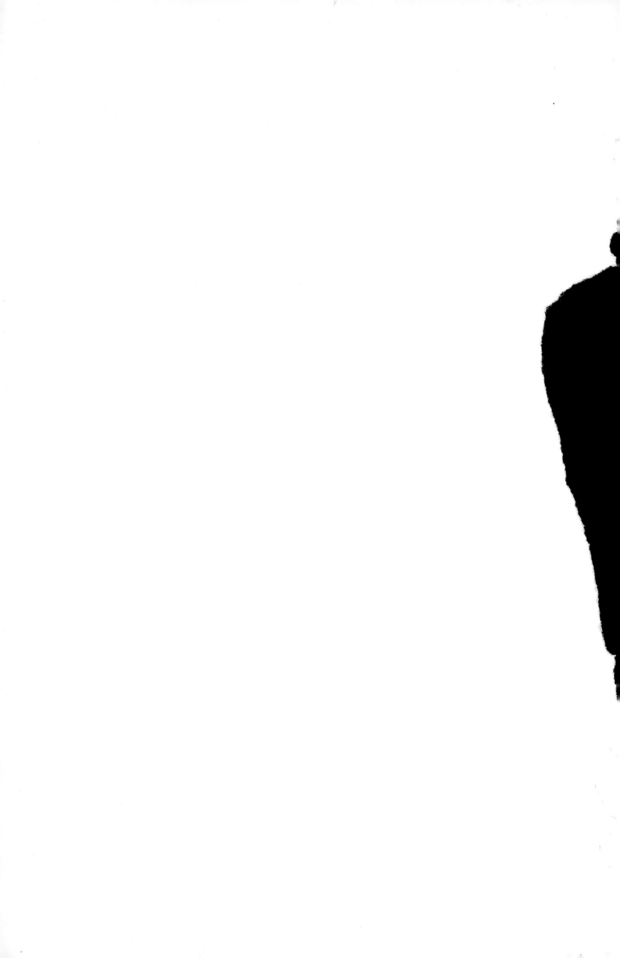